SPECIAL DIET COOKB

MIGRAINE

Dedication
To my GP, Dr Hilary Shaw

NOTE TO READER

Corn has been listed in error on the back cover of the book as a common trigger food. The author would like to emphasize that although each sufferer has their own trigger foods, corn causes problems only in rare instances.

SPECIAL DIET COOKBOOKS
MIGRAINE

CECILIA NORMAN

THORSONS PUBLISHING GROUP

First published 1990

British Library Cataloguing in
Publication Data

Norman, Cecilia
 Migraine special diet cookbook
 1. Migraine sufferers. Food. Recipes
 I. Title
 641.5631

  ISBN 0-7225-2204-5

Published by Thorsons Publishers Limited, Wellingborough, Northamptonshire, NN8 2RQ, England

Typeset by Burns & Smith Ltd., Derby

Printed in Great Britain by The Bath Press, Bath

10 9 8 7 6 5 4 3 2 1

CONTENTS

ACKNOWLEDGEMENTS

Anita Bean BSc
British Dietetic Association
Cadbury Schweppes
Fiona Hunter
Leatherhead Research Association
The Migraine Trust

National Dairy Council
Nutritional Consultative Panel
Queen Charlotte's Hospital
Dr F Clifford Rose, FRCP, Chairman of
the Migraine Trust

FOREWORD

Over a quarter of migraine sufferers believe that their attacks are provoked by some part of their diet. The four 'C's are the commonest, namely, cheese, chocolate, citrus fruits and caffeine, but almost every dietary constituent has been invoked.

Attempts to investigate dietary migraine have not been particularly rewarding. One of the reasons is that trigger factors do not necessarily act in isolation. For example, one patient would have an attack if she was tired and ate pork. If she was tired and did not eat pork, or if she ate pork when she was not tired, she did not have an attack.

This also explains why dietary challenge in a hospital setting often does not provoke the attacks — hence the difficulty in scientifically studying this problem. One study that did produce results was with red wine which almost invariably provoked an attack in those who said they were sensitive to it. And yet an equivalent amount of alcohol (given as vodka — both drinks being disguised) did not provoke the attacks. The hypothesis drawn was that there were chemicals (flavenoid phenols) in the production of red wine from grape skins, etc. which could not be detoxicated by the body because the enzyme necessary (phenolsulphotransferase) was reduced in migraine patients. But these studies are yet to be confirmed.

There is an art as well as a science of medicine: as Plato said,

> Men differ, but they also agree;
> They differ as to what is fleeting but agree as to what is eternal. Difference is in the region of opinion but agreement is the text of truth.

If a trigger factor is found and its avoidance prevents attacks then, clearly, this is much the best way for managing a person with migraine. If the diets in this book help even a fraction of those suffering from migraine, then its publication will serve a valuable purpose.

F CLIFFORD ROSE
Chairman
Migraine Trust

INTRODUCTION

As a migraine sufferer of long standing I have tried a multitude of so-called cures, always hoping to find one to rid me of this tedious complaint. This book has been written out of a heartfelt desire to help fellow sufferers who believe certain foods are contributory to their migraine attacks.

Many do think dietary control is of assistance and each onslaught is to be avoided if at all possible. I trust the guidelines and recipes will be useful.

I am most grateful to all the experts who have advised and counselled me in this endeavour.

ALL ABOUT THE BOOK

This book gives an outline of what migraine is, its factors and how food may affect the likelihood of an attack. With this in mind I have prepared recipes to exclude the more usual 'trigger' foods — i.e., those which are commonly accused of setting off an attack of migraine, like chocolate, cheese and red wine — and also some others that haven't had quite the same bad name.

To ascertain which ingredients may be the cause of *your* migraine, it is important to keep a diary for four to six weeks, listing what you have been doing, where you have been, what you ate and at what time you ate it. You should also note whether the day was particularly stressful or whether it was relaxing. Jot down the weather conditions, how much travelling you did, exercise taken and what time you went to bed. AND most importantly write down if you had a migraine, at what time and how long it lasted on that occasion.

There is a sample diary page at the end of the book. This type of record is better than using odd scraps of paper that may get mislaid.

When the diary is complete, compare the entries carefully and it could well be that you discover the combination of circumstances or causes that bring on an attack for you. If you can detect your own migraine pattern the elimination of particular factors that cause your attacks and the avoidance of your own trigger foods could well materially reduce the frequency of attacks for you. Remember, everybody is an individual — the next person will probably not have the same answer at all.

Most of the ingredients in the recipes in this book can be substituted to suit particular needs to avoid certain foods. In addition the choice of recipes has been designed so that they can be fitted together like a jigsaw to produce a larger variety of meals. For example many of the starters could serve as main courses if combined with other salads or vegetables, and many of the vegetable dishes will be acceptable as main courses.

There is plenty of choice for the vegetarian, who can omit the animal ingredients, and non-vegetarians with larger appetites can usually increase the meat or poultry content without upsetting the balance of the recipe. The chocoholic will find plenty of recipes using permitted carob and there are other sweatmeats to satisfy the sweet-toothed. Eggs — the bugbear of the heart-watcher — do not feature in most of the recipes. Since it is the yolks that contain the cholesterol, when beaten egg would normally be used for coating, egg white will do. Similarly whites can be substituted for most of the yolks when making soufflés.

In my experience few people follow recipes in cookbooks exactly, adding a little of this or that or omitting items they don't personally fancy — but if they do this too liberally they cannot complain if the recipe then doesn't work! However, in this book there is plenty of scope for alteration so hopefully you can go ahead and cook with those alternatives with complete confidence. The recipes have been worked out in both metric and imperial (and also American) measures. These are not necessarily interchangeable so work with only one set in each recipe. Standard measuring spoons have been used and all spoonsful should be level.

A key to the recipes appears on page 32. **Economy tip:** In recipes where safflower oil is listed as an ingredient, sunflower oil can be substituted if preferred. It is lower in polyunsaturated fats, but is generally cheaper.

MIGRAINE — WHAT IS IT?

One in ten people have migraine or have had it at one time or another during their lives. The malady has been recognized since 400 BC and affects 5 per cent of the world's population — and these are mostly women. There are, according to The Migraine Trust, at least 10 million sufferers in the U.K. alone. Sadly all too many families include a migraine victim. The unfortunate person is not the only sufferer as it affects the whole family.

Migraine headaches occur as a result of a combination of factors, including stress, fatigue, relief or relaxation. Stuffy atmospheres — particularly from too many smoking in a confined space — hunger, and food intolerances are further causes. It is a combination of two or more of these that usually precipitates an attack. I am often taken by surprise when, after a period of enormous stress without a migraine on the horizon, I go away for a weekend and after twenty four hours of relaxation, I find myself no longer able to enjoy myself and spend most of the time on the hotel bed.

Each person is different in chemical, hormonal and psychological make-up. As there are so many potential reasons for an attack, so there are several remedies. For you, one or perhaps a combination is right, whereas for others, none of these would be any value at all. This book is for those who find that their headaches are triggered by various foods, which if consumed in anything more than minimal amounts, can tip the chemical balance when other precipitate conditions are also present.

Migraine is not just an ordinary headache. It is an unbearable throbbing accompanied by other unpleasant symptoms. The agony can be excruciating, it makes you feel abjectly unhappy, and it has a nasty habit of ruining many a happy occasion.

Certain other types of headache also produce equally unpleasant effects. These include tension headaches or those which may be indications of more acute conditions. The only other type to be mentioned here is the 'cluster' headache which occurs on consecutive days at infrequent intervals. They start at identical exact times each day, usually in the early hours of the morning so that it is impossible to sleep through them. There may be a feeling of bruising numbness on the bridge of the nose and discomfort from the sinuses on the same side of the face. These attacks usually clear up within an hour or two. These headaches may often be triggered by alcohol.

Migraine has previously been categorized as 'classical' or 'common' but these are now more often known as migraine with or without aura. The only difference between these two major types is that migraine with aura involves the awareness of flashing lights or impaired vision before the onset of an attack. Some people say it is like looking through a net curtain, while others see broken or dancing images. A migraine can start with dramatic suddenness, but the first signs may appear up to twenty four hours beforehand as in my experience.

Common or migraine without aura is the more prevalent and there are usually no pre-attack symptoms. Some sufferers have an aversion to light and sound and the patient may feel very sick. In both types of migraine retching or vomiting can occur and the severity of attack is identical. It doesn't really matter which category of migraine yours comes into, for the fact remains it is still a migraine and it is devastating.

During migraine the blood vessels in the brain are distended. This is caused by chemical changes which are due to an imbalance of proteins and amino acids in the body. Really no one has yet discovered why migraine occurs, but it is understood that there is always a combination of factors.

The poor person concerned may find coherent speech difficult and appear somewhat detached, feel very cold and even shivery, and in the very early stages puff and blow, emitting loud sighs as if short of air and press the hand over one eye or one side of the temple in an effort to suppress the pain. Irritability, short temper or conversely a feeling of immense well-being, exhilaration and unusual bursts of energy are among the warning signs. An unquenchable thirst or sudden desire to binge on chocolate, cheese or olives could predict an attack. Some people have an earache or notice a numbness or neuralgic ache in the arm or down one side of the face and very often a tiny gland at the base of the neck may feel enlarged or tender.

Whatever the signs or symptoms, this is the time to take all possible precautions to pre-empt the attack and alleviate the pain. Once the headache has set in, the sufferer can expect to retire to bed for anything from a few hours to a couple of days with the pain sometimes so intense that sleep is impossible. I find a cold dampened face cloth or large folded handkerchief pressed on to the most painful part of my face (usually my eye) can help dull the agony.

Surprising though it may seem, once an attack has passed, the memory of this recent trauma disappears completely. I am always comforted by the thought that you don't die of migraine. I live opposite one of the big London hospitals and I can see the lights in the wards if I am able to look across from my bed during one of my attacks. I say to myself how lucky I am to be here on my own bed and know that in a few hours I will be up and the migraine will be over.

THE MIGRAINE TYPE

Migraine affects people in all walks of life, from all classes, colours and creeds and in most geographical areas. People of all ages are susceptible and although it is more prevalent in women, neither sex escapes. This is probably because of hormonal and environmental circumstances. For example, mothers who stay at home to look after their children rarely manage to have a few minutes to themselves to relax; the menstrual cycle probably has a strong connection and heredity plays a large part — in my family it has passed from my mother to me and then on to my daughter and now her daughter is showing the first signs of migraine tendency.

If a personality type can be identified, it is likely to be someone who is a worrier, a perfectionist and a meticulous and ambitious person. He or she may be in a position of authority, carrying considerable responsibility, or be in a creative role such as a writer or artist. This is equally true of the conscientious secretary or the shop floor foreman. Those with particularly stressful jobs seem to succumb to bouts of migraine which occur during their leisure hours. As I have already explained, migraine is more likely to occur at weekends or during the first few days of a holiday. On the other hand it rarely happens just at the moment you are going for a job interview or are hyped up to make that important speech. So long as the adrenalin is flowing, migraine attacks seem to be held at bay. I am not at all certain if intense and strung-up people can ever completely relax. If they could find time for regular relaxation might they not be able to reduce the incidence of attacks? It is so difficult to change one's basic make-up and it is certain that after finishing a period of relaxing, you return to worrying immediately. I find structured meditation helps as this requires that you devote two half-hour periods to it each day. The mind may fiercely resist, but the very fact of having to sit still for a prescribed period wears down its stubborness.

Children and migraine

Children *can* suffer from migraine but parents do not always realize this, particularly if they are not sufferers themselves. Perhaps the child is assumed to be just off-colour or simply malingering and doesn't want to go to school. Frequent complaints of feeling sick or having a tummy ache, with or without actual vomiting, may well be symptoms that here is a young migraine sufferer. Other signs may be trouble with seeing properly (although the child may well not mention it), or the youngster is irritable with yawning, tiredness and loss of energy. While car sickness may not be due to migraine, children who get migraine will be prone to travel sickness.

Fortunately children's migraine attacks seldom have the intensity of those suffered by an adult. Except for individuals destined to be affected throughout their lives, children usually grow out of it on reaching puberty.

If one or other of the parents is a migraine sufferer, it will naturally be possible to cope so much more understandingly with the child's disability. Too much TV, prolonged play in bright sunlight or junk foods are likely triggers, whilst hunger or bad dreams are other indications of causes in the young. It is well worth taking your child to your GP to check if it is migraine or some sign of another illness. If migraine is then confirmed, the single act of cutting out chocolate may be sufficient to change the pattern. Watch what and when your child is eating. So many children eat junk foods that their intake of monosodium glutamate or the preservative sodium nitrite might be excessive and these are food triggers. Tell your child he will never die of or from migraine and that it won't develop into anything worse. A child's imagination is unbounded and you never know what terrible fears he may be suffering each time he gets an attack, and indeed fear may bring one on.

Factors that bring on an attack

The Migraine Clinic lists at least five major areas:-

Physical	– fatigue; over-exertion; relaxation
Psychological	– depression; worry; shock; anxiety
Medical	– contraceptives; blood pressure; menstruation
Outside factors	– loud noises; glaring lights; discos and flashing lights; TV; computer screens
Diet	– consumption of alcohol; trigger foods; strong smells

CHOICE OF TREATMENT

The wisest move to make when you first think that you have a migraine is to go to your doctor. He or she will be able to determine if this is a true migraine or simply a bad headache with a tummy upset. A couple of aspirins taken right at the beginning may well do the trick. If a simple treatment does not succeed, you then have to decide whether you wish to follow the path of conventional medicine, whether you believe that complementary medicine will be more beneficial or whether a combination of both may give the best results. Ergotomine is prescribed in extreme cases but this is a dangerous drug and can only be taken in controlled amounts. If taken at the wrong time it can make the patient feel temporarily worse.

The conventional paths could lead to referral by your GP to the Migraine Clinic. The Migraine Trust based at Great Ormond Street will send you all the necessary information about the treatments available at the Clinic and tell you about the success that can be obtained. The trouble is that they really advise you to go to see them when you are suffering from an attack and, of course, this is the last thing you want to do at such a time. However, if you can face up to it, their diagnostic ability and remedies are most helpful.

Alternative or complementary medicine includes herbs, yoga, hypnosis, acupuncture, aromatherapy, chiropractic, homoeopathy and osteopathy. The most well-known herbal remedy is feverfew. This can either be taken in green leaf form by eating a feverfew sandwich (I personally mix it with lettuce leaves which I find has a definite benefit) or it can be taken in pill form. Yoga is one of the examples of relaxation exercise which can be of help. Since migraine can so often be brought on by anxiety or stress, any relieving of tensions must be of assitance. Meditation practised regularly disciplines the mind and so de-stresses it. Similarly hypnosis can help to overcome symptoms of stress, and self-hypnosis, under guidance, might well help to reduce stress-induced migraine. Acupuncture is the oldest unorthodox therapy. It is well worth a try and if you are afraid of needles, there is now a less scary method of application. Aromatherapy consists of a wonderfully relaxing massage using heavenly perfumes and natural oils. I have fallen into a deep remedial sleep during an ordinary beauty treatment and aromatherapy is undoubtedly more luxurious than that. In any event the periods of complete rest during these treatments — or in fact any of the others in the complementary medicine field — are always beneficial. A chiropractor will work on the pressure points of the neck, head and spine to try and unravel taut muscles and remove the odd nodule. Although some osteopathic treatments may work, they can themselves initiate a migraine attack, particularly at the beginning of a series of treatments. But it is usual, over a period of time, for the treatment to reduce the frequency of attacks.

All these alternative medicine treatments are normally of little value if you have no faith in their ability to work for you. On the other hand if you have a deep conviction that a particular treatment will and does work for you, its success rate is bound to be higher, because of the reduction in stress that the patient experiences while undergoing the treatment and from the mental serenity it subsequently induces.

Whatever your choice as to medical treatment, it should go hand in glove with care over your diet. Food and drink are the main ingredients of body maintenance and without them we would not be able to exist. Good sensible nutrition has never been more uppermost in our minds than is the case in the present day and we are all diet-aware. The migraine and allergy sufferer needs to be even more alert about this than most and it is vital to find out which ingredients affect you. With care you may be able to escape the terrible scourge of migraine, the fear of which hangs over you like an ominous dark cloud.

Doing without food, slimming and fasting, missing a meal because you simply have no time, or leaving a long gap between the last snack at night and a late late breakfast are bad news for the migraine person. While others may just develop a headache — and bad breath — a quick bite will make them feel better almost immediately. The migraine person, on the other hand, having started the headache, will find that it is too late and will already be in the middle of another attack.

During a migraine, the thought of eating is abhorrent, although I find my lettuce and feverfew sandwich is acceptable and sometimes actually helps. When you sense an attack coming on, have a proper hot meal and not just a snack. Don't try to keep going — take ten to fifteen minutes to sit alone in a dimly lit room and close your eyes. That small amount of relaxation can make all the difference.

Low blood sugar may precipitate an attack and this is another reason for eating. It does not have to be a high calorie meal and certainly it should not be a rich one. Generally plainly cooked food is the ideal. Try not to let too much time elapse between eating. If you are accustomed to eating at about 6 o'clock, yet are dining at 8, the usual pattern is destroyed and the gap is too long, so have something to eat, even if it's only a couple of dry biscuits before you leave the house.

DIET AND MIGRAINE

A migraine is not caused by one factor alone. In normal day-to-day life a piece of chocolate or cheese will have no adverse effect, but on a day which has been stressful, where there has been no possibility of having a proper meal, and if fatigued and travelling perchance in a hot stuffy car — perhaps with a brightly lit tunnel on the way home — that piece of chocolate may well be the straw that breaks the camel's back.

Chronic or frequent migraine sufferers will try to take precautions against acquiring another migraine and so will exclude any likely triggers from their diet. It is possible that specific foods in addition to lack of food, can trigger an attack. This may be because certain chemicals in food may affect the blood vessels, most likely in the brain, causing fluctuations in the blood pressure. Adverse reaction to certain foods or ingredients — one must distinguish this carefully from food allergy — are said to start migraine attacks in a large number of people. Naturally every person is different and any particular substance can cause a reaction in an individual, but for those who consider their migraine attacks are triggered by food, the main categories are:

1. Chocolate
2. Cheese
3. Dairy products
4. Citrus fruits
5. Wheat
6. Alcohol — particularly red wine

These are the categories I am concerned with in the book and which I will, in the recipes, provide alternatives and substitutes for or alert you to their presence. Absence of the main triggers are listed at the bottom of each recipe. Substitute ingredients are noted where appropriate.

Dr Edda Hanington, author of *The Headache Book* and *Migraine*, found in a scientific survey of 500 patients that 74 per cent were convinced that chocolate was the culprit, 47 per cent cheese and dairy products, 30 per cent fruit (in particular citrus fruits), closely followed by alcohol 25 per cent. Eighteen per cent thought vegetables and fried fatty foods were responsible and below these came tea and coffee at 15 per cent, meat (especially pork) 14 per cent and seafood 10 per cent.

Dr Hanington stated that it was apparent that various chemicals entered the system via food and these chemicals in the bloodstream can affect the blood vessels, which cause the throbbing sensation in a migraine headache. The culprits are nearly always one or other of the amines. Chocolate has betaphenlethylamine, alcohol has hystamine, cheese has tyramine (so do pickled herrings, but I have never heard of a complaint about them!), citrus fruits have octopamine. People whose systems do not have enough enzymes to discourage the action on their bodies of these amines, may have as a result a surfeit of these protein particles which can thereby fuel the migraine.

Experimental work continues, specifically at Queen Charlotte's Hospital in London, to scientifically examine possible dietary triggers. Remember the diary I suggested earlier — you may well be able to pinpoint your particular *bêtes noires*. The stimulus for your attacks, if caused by a trigger substance, may be any one of the potential food hazards or it could be all of them and certain others as well, such as monosodium glutamate, yeast extract, potatoes, nuts, fudge, olives, yoghurt, double cream, strong tea or coffee, pork, sausages and other meat products which contain preservatives. These have all had the reputation of being some person's downfall at some time or another.

FOOD SUBSTITUTES

The body's tolerance to a chemical build-up which precipitates a migraine in susceptible people is limited. Sufferers may prefer to play safe and restrict or exclude certain foods.

Alcohol

There is no evidence that alcohol *per se* causes migraine attacks to develop. However, we all know that too much drink can cause a headache, and a hangover can seem remarkably similar to a light attack of migraine. Wine certainly contains histamine which occurs as the result of the fermentation process. Experiments undoubtedly conclude that red wine is the biggest culprit, as rosé and white wines are more acceptable with less bad after-effects. I also believe that a good vintage red can be less troublesome than plonk, so one wonders if the tannin in less mature reds could be the trigger for some — the early removal of the pith and pips from the mush when producing white and rosé wines could be the saving grace for those wines.

The aroma hanging over the French countryside when the vigneroles bring in the crop of grapes to the co-operatives for the vendange is extremely heady. One might feel that more than a few deep breaths could bring on an instant migraine. Those with a great liking for the taste of the grape might do well to settle for the less romantic grape juice which can be attractively served but which has none of the offending contents.

I would venture to suggest one tip which I have found surprisingly effective. Never drink wine when thirsty — always quench your thirst with water. At the table drink some plain or sparkling water before even taking a sip of the wine. Ask for a glass of water when dining out in addition to your glass of wine and drink from each glass alternately. Certainly in France many people actually mix water with their wine and this dilution will lessen the bad effects.

Cheese

Substitutes can be found for most recipe ingredients but one of the most common and basic foodstuffs — cheese — seems to be a major culprit and sadly has no natural flavour replacement. However there is no need to eschew all cheeses since many contain only minimal amounts of tyramine (which is one of the amines produced by changes caused by the amino acid, tyrosine). Tyramine levels rise during fermentation so that Roquefort, Gorgonzola and other blue-veined cheeses come at the top of the forbidden list. Mature Cheddar is undesirable as it contains 1466 milligrams per gram. Gruyère has 516, Brie 150 and Camembert ranges from 20–86 per gram, depending on the ripeness. Cottage cheese has a negligible amount and few fresh soft unmatured cheeses will be likely to be responsible for inducing an attack. Cheese-lovers can reduce the tyramine content by settling for a Welsh Rarebit made with a combination of curd and a modicum of Cheshire Cheese. Soufflés need not be totally banned provided the cheese chosen is low in tyramine. Use nuts, oats, coarse cornmeal or breadcrumbs for crusty brown toppings and if you have previously enjoyed grilled halloumi, try grilled, smoked or marinated tofu. Part of the secret is to eat cheese in small amounts only and so while a Ploughman's lunch is undesirable, often being served with a 75g to 100g/3 oz to 4 oz portion of mature Cheddar, a reasonable serving of cheese sauce, comprising 10g/½ oz young Gouda will not be deleterious.

Chocolate

Chocolate contains only small quantities of tyramine which was always thought to be the most potent ingredient. But it also has other amines, histamine and betaphenlethylamine, making it highly inadvisable to eat it at the same meal as cheese. Refuse the cheese board *and* the after dinner mints if you are even slightly at risk. Caffeine is also present in chocolate, so you may well be advised to decide against the coffee as well.

Unfortunately the chocolate 'addict' finds it impossible to consume only one small piece and inevitably ends up with an even greater craving. Chocolate, for those whom it affects, is most definitely *out*. Sadly it cannot be replaced by cocoa, because this is the substance from which chocolate is made and so has all the same unwelcome amines.

However all is not lost, because carob, having a related flavour, yet being in no way connected with the cocoa bean, is a most acceptable replacement. Carob pods grow on trees of the same name and proliferate in Mediterranean countries. Visitors to Cyprus cannot have failed to see them. The pods grow on the female trees and are about the size of broad beans. They start off green but then turn to brown. After the seeds are removed for other uses the pods are roasted and milled. Carob in powder form is a finer and more fly-away texture than cocoa and must be kept in very dry conditions to avoid lumpiness. To make carob bars and chips, vegetable fat and lecithin are added. These bars are easily melted in the same way as chocolate and perform the same function, which is indeed a comfort to the chocolate lover. The only slight disadvantage is that it has a matt appearance when set. This can be remedied by the addition of a few drops of fresh vegetable oil. Carob contains none of the unacceptable amines and no caffeine. Naturally sweet, carob needs much less additional sweetening, but it can also be obtained with added sweetener. In cooking, substitute 2 tablespoons of carob powder for 25g/1 oz chocolate. Carob bars and drops vary in their content. Sometimes they contain milk (but this can be non-dairy) and greater or lesser amounts of sweetening. In cookery this does not vary the result.

Sweet-toothed people may well be content with other chocolate substitutes and so will settle for sweetmeats such as fudge and toffee. The sweetmeat section is specially designed for them.

Citrus fruits

Citrus fruits contain Vitamin C so it is important to include other Vitamin C-rich foods in your diet if you have to exclude citrus fruits. Green leafy vegetables are good sources. Vitamin C powder can be added to most dishes and will also replace the chemical reaction in cookery that is the purpose served by lemon juice in so many recipes. Good quality malt or cider vinegar can replace lemon juice in sauces and salad dressings and is also a helpful raising agent in cakes when heavier flours than wheat flours are called for.

Milk cream and butter

Dairy produce is defined as foods derived from cow's milk. There is a separate heading devoted to cheese alone, which is probably the most important trigger food, because of the tyramine development during the manufacturing process. Other dairy produce does not contain tyramine to any extent.

Although goats are bovine creatures, it seems that goats' milk and yoghurt made from goats' milk may be acceptable to those whose intolerance stems from the size of the fat in globules in milk. These are smaller in goats' milk and so are more easily assimilated. (However, goats' milk is not routinely pasteurized and lacks folic acid, necessary for infant nutrition.) Lactose intolerance is uncommon. So is cows' milk allergy which derives from the proteins it contains. The incidence is so low it is most unlikely to have any effect on migraine.

Vegetarians who make up 3 per cent of the population of the U.K. may consume milk and milk products provided that no animal rennet is used in cheese-making and no gelatine is added to yoghurt. For vegans all dairy produce is forbidden.

Luckily there are plenty of available substitutes, including plant and nut milks, yoghurt and non-dairy cream (which is made from mainly water, vegetable oil and sugar). Soya milk is readily obtainable either sweetened or unsweetened, while nut milk can be made by pulverizing the nuts and leaving them to soak in water before straining. Coconut milk is good in sweet dishes and is also acceptable in those savoury recipes where the strong flavour of the coconut will not mask the more subtle flavours.

Non-dairy cream can be whipped and although it does not have the flavour of fresh cream, a textural difference is undetectable.

There are various butter substitutes available, including soya margarine, vegetable fats and polyunsaturated margarines. These latter may contain whey. Oil should always be fresh and the mono and polyunsaturated kinds are better for health. Sunflower oil has practically no flavour and is high in polyunsaturates. Corn oil is mildly flavoured, but nut oils, such as hazelnut and walnut, and seed oils such as sesame, have a pronounced taste. Olive oil is thicker and is a mono-unsaturate. Its flavour will depend on where it comes from and whether it is a virgin oil (almost green in colour) or a second pressing. These cheaper late pressings produce a paler appearance. Olive oil may be too heavy to use in cake-making, but it is ideal in savoury dishes and salads.

Dripping, which is non-dairy (and of course also non-vegetarian) can often be substituted in cooking, but this does add cholesterol unnecessarily.

Wheat

A sizeable proportion of migraine people say that they find wheat to be a trigger food. This may not necessarily be because it contains gluten. But if having omitted wheat from the diet the substitution of rye, barley, buckwheat and oat flour appears to bring on a migraine, if may signify a gluten intolerance. However oats are considered to be less of a problem and are nutritionally valuable, so should not be summarily excluded. There is plenty of choice as far as flours are concerned but to produce light well-risen baked goods and in particular bread, there must be a proportion of wheat flour.

Flours made from nuts, cereals, pulses and vegetables, and starches such as arrowroot and cornflour, are all easily obtainable, and one of my all-round favourites, gram flour is on sale at all Indian-type grocers. Soy bean flour and products made from the soy bean such as tempeh and tofu can be obtained from health food shops or specialist Japanese or Chinese emporia and some operate a mail-order system. Health shops stock all the usual brown rice, potato (farina) and nut flours and also sell tapioca, oatmeal, millet and a variety of others. It is fascinating and worthwhile to experiment and to this end, I am including some notes on their functions in cookery.

1. ARROWROOT is made from the tubers of a West Indian plant.
It contains practically no protein.
It helps lighten wheatless cakes but must not replace more than 50 per cent wheat flour. Has good thickening properties. Use in equal quantities to replace cornflour.
For a pouring sauce use 1 level tablespoon to 300ml/½ pint/1⅓ cupsful liquid, adding more for a thicker sauce. The longer the sauce is cooked the thinner it becomes, so that it is better to add the arrowroot dissolved in a little cold water towards the end of cooking. Should the sauce need to be reheated it will be necessary to add a little more blended arrowroot when raising the heat to boiling point. Remember to stir continuously.
It is useful for coating prior to frying or roasting.

2. CORNFLOUR is made from maize.
It has a slightly higher protein content than arrowroot and produces glossier sauces and is less lumpy when cool. In cakemaking it produces a light crumb. Can be used to replace up to 25 per cent wheat flour.

3. BROWN RICE FLOUR is made from brown rice and is gluten free.
It has a mild flavour but does produce an off-white tint to sauces.
It is not recommended for coating, but is useful in biscuits and pastry.

To use for thickening, increase amount by 20 per cent when replacing wheat flour.

Sauces will thicken and become smooth on standing. Reheat as necessary.

Cakes will be too dry unless other flours or nuts are included so substitute 25 per cent of the brown rice flour with ground almonds. Add stewed or fresh fruit, grated carrot or courgettes and a little oil to prevent cakes becoming dry.

Replace wheat flour with 50 per cent oat flour or fine oatmeal and 50 per cent brown rice flour.

In most recipes replace 100g/4 oz wheat flour with 90g/3½ oz brown rice flour.

4. BUCKWHEAT FLOUR is made from the seeds of a fruit which are finely milled and has a significant gluten content.

Most available buckwheat flour is made from roasted seeds and generally is too strong and powerfully flavoured to be used on its own.

It is more acceptable when mixed with cornflour. Because of its pronounced flavour it is unsuitable for thickening, but can be useful for coating savoury foods prior to frying. Items so coated must be fried at a lower temperature to ensure that browning does not occur before the food is thoroughly cooked. This flour is used for Brittany pancakes and Russian blinis.

5. POTATO FLOUR (also called farina) is made from cooked potato.

It is white and flavourless and must be kept in a cold place as its shelf-life is limited.

Its gelling properties are good. It can be used for thickening, but only add small quantities, blending it first with cold liquid. Dishes thickened with potato flour should be served hot or may be lumpy when cool. Browns well in baking, but is less efficient as a coating for fried items.

It is a good all-round ingredient which can also be used in biscuits and cakes, not necessarily in conjunction with wheat flour, but mixed with other flours.

6. OAT FLOUR is finely ground oatmeal containing a certain amount of gluten.

It can always be prepared at home from fine, medium, coarse oatmeal or porridge oats. Excellent for baking, it has a nutty and appetizing flavour. It is a useful ingredient in pastry-making and is the main ingredient in flapjacks. Substitute oat flour or fine oatmeal for wheat flour, but the results will be even better if up to 50 per cent rice flour or arrowroot is included. The thickening qualities of oatmeal are obvious to anyone in the habit of making porridge and in common with other kinds of meal, further thickening occurs if mixtures are given a standing time. Use about the same weight as wheat flour but bear in mind that the resulting sauces will have a grey tinge.

Use medium oatmeal as a coating for grilling or frying and as a topping for crisp fruity puddings.

7. SOYA FLOUR is made from the soya bean.

In baking it may be used in place of 25 per cent of wheat flour but cakes baked solely from soya flour have a noticeably poor rise. When used half and half with arrowroot or cornflour, the finished item is moist and has a good texture.

Adequate for coating food to be fried but rather poor if used for thickening.

8. CHICK PEA FLOUR

Has a mild flavour and gives sauces a yellow tone. It is not good for coating but first class for thickening. Especially useful in stews where the colour and flavour are masked.

As a baking substitute it is best mixed in a 25 per cent ratio with other flours or in 50 per cent ratio with ground nuts.

9. GRAM FLOUR is made from differing varieties of pulses or beans.

Besam flour is made from split peas and is my favourite for making batters, requiring only cold water to adhere. Add spices and a little salt and pepper and use to make little dropped pancakes or as a coating for savoury fritters. Excellent for binding.

Besam flour is used together with curry spices, turmeric and chopped onions as the recipe for onion bhajias. The joy of besam flour is that it is non-dairy and no eggs are needed, making it suitable for vegetarians and vegans as well as everyone else. Various Indian sweetmeats are made from other types of pulse, including ground green lentils, also known as mung beans.

Key to recipes:

C   – Citrus free
D   – Dairy free
MSG – Monosodium Glutamate free
Veg   – Vegetarian
Vegan – Vegan
W   – Wheat free

Variations to this code appear
occasionally on individual recipes.

BREAKFASTS

Breakfast Drop Pancakes

Makes 6 to 8
Serves 4

UK

40g/1½ oz cornflour
1 egg
1 tablespoon milk
generous pinch bicarbonate of soda
pinch salt
pinch sugar
pinch ground cinnamon [optional]
1 tablespoon oil

US

⅓ cup cornstarch
1 egg
1 tablespoon milk
generous pinch baking soda
pinch salt
pinch sugar
pinch ground cinnamon [optional]
1 tablespoon oil

1. Put the cornflour (cornstarch) in a bowl or measuring jug and beat in the egg and milk.
2. Stir in the remaining ingredients except the oil.
3. Lightly oil and heat a non-stick frying pan (skillet) and put 3 separate tablespoons of the batter, well spaced out, on to the hot pan.
4. Cook until lightly browned underneath, then flip the pancakes over to cook the other sides. Stir remaining batter and cook another batch of pancakes.
5. Serve with grilled (broiled) tomatoes, kipper fillets, poached eggs, sausages or maple syrup or jam.

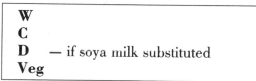

W
C
D — if soya milk substituted
Veg

Creamy Mushrooms on Golden Hash Browns

Serves 4

UK

25g/1 oz butter
225g/8 oz button mushrooms, rinsed, wiped dry and finely sliced
4 tablespoons cornflour or flour
300ml/½ pint milk
salt
freshly ground black pepper
1 recipe Golden Hash Browns [see page 88]

US

2½ tablespoons butter
4 cups button mushrooms, rinsed, wiped dry and finely sliced
4 tablespoons cornstarch or flour
1¼ cups milk
salt
freshly ground black pepper
1 recipe Golden Hash Browns [see page 88]

1. Melt the butter in a medium saucepan, stir in the mushrooms and cook gently until tender.
2. Draw pan away from the heat and thoroughly blend in cornflour (cornstarch) or flour.
3. Stir in milk and season with salt and pepper.
4. Replace pan over medium heat, bring to boil, stirring continuously, then continue cooking for 3 to 4 minutes, still stirring.
5. Divide freshly cooked hash browns into four wedges and top with the mushroom mixture.

W — if cornflour (cornstarch) used	
C	
D — if vegetable margarine and milk are substituted	
Veg	

Grape and Kiwi Nectar

Serves 4

UK

450g/1 lb red seedless grapes
2 kiwi fruit
4–6 teaspoons icing sugar

US

1 pound seedless grapes
2 kiwi fruit
4–6 teaspoons icing sugar

1. Wash the grapes and remove any stalks. Pat dry on kitchen paper.
2. Peel the kiwi fruit, cut in half and remove 4 thin centre slices for decoration.
3. Place the fruit in a juice extractor or liquidize in a blender.
4. Pour through a strainer into a wide-necked jug, pressing the pulp with a wooden spoon to extract all the juice. Stir in the sugar until dissolved.
5. Float the reserved kiwi slices on the juice and refrigerate until well chilled.

> **C**
> **Vegan**

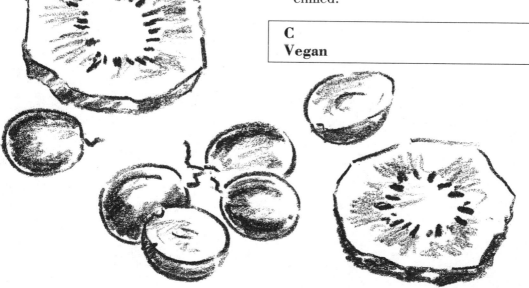

Kedgeree

Serves 4

UK

2 tablespoons sunflower oil
1 small onion, (chopped)
175g/6 oz long grain rice, boiled
350g/12 oz smoked haddock fillet,
   skinned and flaked
2 hard-boiled eggs, chopped
2 tablespoons chopped fresh parsley
cayenne
freshly ground black pepper
paprika

US

2 tablespoons safflower oil
1 small onion, chopped
1 cup long grain rice, boiled
12 ounces smoked haddock fillet,
   skinned and flaked
2 hard-cooked eggs, chopped
2 tablespoons chopped fresh parsley
cayenne
freshly ground black pepper
paprika

1. Heat the oil and gently fry onion until soft.
2. Add rice, fish, egg, parsley, a shake of cayenne and a shake of black pepper. Reheat over low heat.
3. Turn mixture into a warmed serving dish and garnish with a few shakes of paprika.

W
C
D
Veg — if 175g/6 oz/⅔ cup smoked tofu strips substituted for fish

Muesli

Serves 10 to 12

UK

225g/8 oz quick porridge oats
25g/1 oz oat bran
2 tablespoons sunflower seeds, toasted
50g/2 oz shelled hazelnuts, roasted and
  chopped
50g/2 oz dried apple rings, chopped
3 stoned prunes, chopped
2 dried pear halves, chopped
1 tablespoon raisins
1 tablespoon sultanas
1 tablespoon soft brown sugar

US

2 cups quick porridge oats
¼ cup oat bran
2 tablespoons sunflower seeds, toasted
½ cup shelled hazelnuts, roasted and
  chopped
3 tablespoons dried apple rings, chopped
3 pitted prunes, chopped
2 dried pear halves, chopped
1 tablespoon raisins
1 tablespoon golden seedless raisins
1 tablespoon soft brown sugar

1. Mix all the ingredients together and
   store for up to 2 weeks in a tightly
   lidded plastic container in the
   refrigerator.

Serve with milk, yoghurt, soya milk, non-
dairy cream or fruit juice.

W
D
C
Vegan

Melon and Ginger Juice

UK

1 ripe honeydew melon
6-mm/¼-inch thick slice fresh ginger root
2–3 tablespoons clear honey

US

1 ripe honeydew melon
¼-inch thick slice fresh ginger root
2–3 tablespoons clear honey

1. Divide the melon into 4 wedges, remove the seeds, then cut the flesh away from the peel.
2. Cut the flesh into chunks and liquidize with the ginger root and honey.
3. Pour through a strainer into a wide-necked jug, pressing the pulp with a wooden spoon to extract all the juice.
4. Refrigerate until well chilled.

C
Vegan

SOUPS

Beetroot Soup

Serves 4 to 5
Makes 1 litre/1¾ pints/4 cups

UK

175g/6 oz raw or cooked beetroot, peeled and grated
1 medium carrot, scraped and grated
1 small potato, peeled and grated
1 teaspoon cider vinegar
450ml/¾ pint well-flavoured stock
300ml/½ pint tomato juice
1 teaspoon sugar
salt
freshly ground black pepper
150ml/¼ pint non-dairy cream

US

1½ cups raw or cooked beet, peeled and grated
1 medium carrot, scraped and grated
1 small potato, peeled and grated
1 teaspoon cider vinegar
2 cups well-flavored stock
1¼ cups tomato juice
1 teaspoon sugar
salt
freshly ground black pepper
⅔ cup non-dairy cream

1. Put the beetroot, carrot, potato, vinegar, stock, tomato juice and sugar in a large saucepan.
2. Bring to the boil, cover and simmer for 35 minutes to 45 minutes. Season with salt and pepper to taste.
3. Stir in the cream and remove pan from the heat.
4. Serve hot or cold.

If a smoother soup is preferred, it may be puréed in the blender.

| W |
| C |
| D |
| Vegan |

Brussels Sprouts Soup

Serves 6

UK

450g/1 lb Brussels sprouts, trimmed and
 washed
1 small onion, peeled and quartered
1.2 litres/2 pints well-flavoured stock
3 tablespoons sunflower oil
40g/1½ oz flour
300ml/½ pint milk
salt
pepper

US

1 pound Brussels sprouts, trimmed and
 washed
1 small onion, peeled and quartered
5 cups well-flavored stock
3 tablespoons safflower oil
6 tablespoons flour
1¼ cups milk
salt
pepper

1. Put the sprouts, onion and stock in a large saucepan and simmer until soft.
2. Blend to a purée. Mix oil, flour and milk together.
3. Combine purée and flour mixture in the large saucepan and cook over medium heat, stirring continuously until soup thickens. Cook for 2 more minutes, still stirring. Season with salt and pepper if needed.
4. Serve hot.

C
W — if 3 tablespoons potato flour is substituted for the flour
Veg

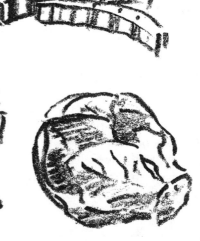

Cantonese Soup

Serves 4

UK

900ml/1½ pints chicken stock
100g/4 oz boned chicken breast,
   shredded
2.5-cm/1-inch strip red pepper, thinly
   sliced
50g/2 oz bamboo shoots, thinly sliced
50g/2 oz button mushrooms, quartered
50g/2 oz beansprouts, rinsed
25g/1 oz cooked rice
salt
freshly ground black pepper

US

3¾ cups chicken stock
1 cup boned chicken breast, shredded
1-inch strip red pepper, thinly sliced
1 cup bamboo shoots, thinly sliced
1 cup button mushrooms, quartered
1 cup beansprouts, rinsed
1 tablespoon cooked rice
salt
freshly ground black pepper

1. Put the stock and shredded chicken in a large saucepan.
2. Bring to the boil, then simmer for 10 minutes.
3. Stir in pepper strips, bamboo shoots and mushrooms. Simmer for 10 minutes or until chicken and vegetables are cooked.
4. Add beansprouts and rice. Bring to the boil, then season to taste with salt and pepper.

> **W**
> **C**
> **MSG**

Cream of Tomato Soup

Serves 4 to 6
Makes 850ml/1½ pints/3¾ cups

UK

2 tablespoons sunflower oil
4 tablespoons cornflour
300ml/½ pint milk
1×800g/1 lb 12 oz tin tomatoes
¼ teaspoon chopped basil leaves
generous pinch dried rosemary
generous pinch oregano
salt
freshly ground black pepper
generous pinch sugar

US

2 tablespoons safflower oil
4 tablespoons cornstarch
1¼ cups milk
2×14½ ounce cans tomatoes
¼ teaspoon chopped basil leaves
generous pinch dried rosemary
generous pinch oregano
salt
freshly ground black pepper
generous pinch sugar

1. Combine oil, cornflour and milk in a large saucepan.
2. Cook, stirring continuously over low heat until thickened.
3. Add tomatoes and their juice and the herbs and crush with a fork or potato masher.
4. Add 150ml/¼ pint water. Bring back to boil. Season with salt and pepper and add sugar.
5. Blend soup to a purée. Strain into the saucepan through a nylon sieve.
6. Reheat and serve hot.

W
C
D — if soya milk is substituted
Veg

Home-made Chicken Soup

Makes 2.25 litres/4 pints/10 cups

UK

1 × 1.5kg/3¼ lb chicken, washed and cut
   into 8 pieces
giblets from the chicken
4 carrots, scraped and cut into chunks
2 onions, quartered
12 black peppercorns
salt

US

1 × 3¼ pound chicken, washed and cut
   into 8 pieces
giblets from chicken
4 carrots, scraped and cut into chunks
2 onions, quartered
12 black peppercorns
salt

> **W**
> **C**
> **MSG**

1. Put chicken pieces and giblets in very large saucepan. Cover with cold water and bring to boil.
2. Skim and continue cooking, removing scum until it no longer forms.
3. Add vegetables and peppercorns and season sparingly with salt.
4. Reduce heat, cover and cook gently for 4 hours, topping up with water as necessary.
5. Strain into a large bowl. Pick the chicken meat from the bones and shred finely. Cool meat rapidly and refrigerate as soon as possible.
6. Leave soup to cool, then strain to remove any deposits.
7. Chill until fat forms a solid layer on top.
8. Remove fat, saving it for use in non-dairy dishes if wished.
9. Adjust seasoning.
10. Reheat to boiling point with shredded chicken.

Omit onion if wished. Always re-boil before use. Can be used as chicken stock. Will freeze.

Iced Cucumber Soup

Serves 4
Makes 600ml/1 pint/2½ cups

UK

15g/½ oz butter
1 slice onion, chopped
1 medium cucumber, rinsed and diced
300ml/½ pint well-flavoured chicken
   stock
5–7 tablespoons milk
salt
white pepper
1 level tablespoon chopped chives

US

1¼ tablespoons butter
1 slice onion, chopped
1 medium cucumber, rinsed and diced
1¼ cups well-flavored chicken stock
5–7 tablespoons milk
salt
white pepper
1 level tablespoon chopped chives

1. Put butter and onion in a large saucepan and stir over medium heat for 1 minute.
2. Add cucumber and continue cooking for 2 minutes, stirring gently.
3. Add stock, bring to boil, then reduce heat and cook covered for 15 minutes.
4. Blend to a purée.
5. Add milk and reheat in saucepan to boiling point. [see note below]
6. Pour into bowl, cover and cool. Chill for 2 to 3 hours. Season with salt and pepper before serving.
7. Serve chilled garnished with chopped chives.

For a richer soup, beat 1 egg yolk with 3 tablespoons cream or milk and 3 table-spoons hot soup. Return to saucepan when adding milk, reheat, stirring continuously, to just below boiling point.

W
C
D — if vegetable margarine and
    milk are substituted

Lentil Soup

Serves 4

UK

175g/6 oz red lentils
1.2 litres/2 pints water or stock
1 lean bacon rasher, chopped
1 medium onion, chopped
1 medium carrot, chopped
2 bay leaves
pinch ground cardamom
salt
freshly ground black pepper

US

1 cup red lentils
5 cups water or stock
1 lean bacon rasher, chopped
1 medium onion, chopped
1 medium carrot, chopped
2 bay leaves
pinch ground cardamom
salt
freshly ground black pepper

1. Put all ingredients **except salt and pepper** in a large saucepan.
2. Boil rapidly for ten minutes, then simmer gently for 1 to 1½ hours until lentils are soft.
3. Remove bay leaves. Season to taste with salt and pepper.
4. Purée in the blender or press through a sieve. Add extra water or stock if too thick.
5. Reheat.

Serve sprinkled with chopped parsley or diced wholemeal toast.

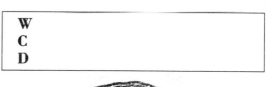

W
C
D

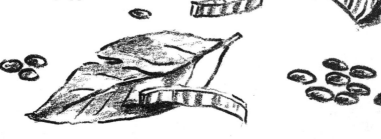

Lettuce Soup

Serves 4

UK

1 round lettuce
salt
4 spring onions, trimmed and sliced
40g/1½ oz butter or margarine
450ml/¾ pint vegetable or chicken stock
pinch sugar
pinch ground mace
450ml/¾ pint milk
pepper

US

1 Bibb lettuce
salt
4 scallions, trimmed and sliced
3¾ tablespoons butter or margarine
2 cups vegetable or chicken stock
pinch sugar
pinch ground mace
2 cups milk
pepper

1. Wash lettuce, separate leaves and remove any thick stems.
2. Place in large saucepan of boiling salted water.
3. Bring back to boil, then simmer for 5 minutes.
4. Drain and finely shred.
5. In same saucepan gently fry spring onions (scallions) in butter for 3 minutes until soft.
6. Add lettuce and stock, sugar and mace.
7. Simmer covered for 15 to 20 minutes.
8. Purée soup and stir in milk. Reheat, then add salt only if needed and pepper to taste.
9. Serve hot.

W
C
Substitute vegetable margarine and milk if wished
Veg

Pumpkin Soup

Serves 4 to 5

UK

1.5kg/3¼ lb pumpkin, deseeded and
   chopped
1 small onion, sliced
600ml/1 pint stock
600ml/1 pink milk
salt
pepper
generous pinch ground nutmeg
3 tablespoons cream
1 tablespoon finely chopped roasted
   hazelnuts

US

3¼ pounds pumpkin, deseeded and
   chopped
1 small onion, sliced
2½ cups stock
2½ cups milk
salt
pepper
generous pinch ground nutmeg
3 tablespoons cream
1 tablespoon finely chopped roasted
   hazelnuts

1. Combine pumpkin, onion and stock in a large saucepan.
2. Simmer covered for 45 minutes to 1 hour until tender. Sieve or purée the soup. Add milk and reheat to steaming point, stirring continuously.
3. Season with salt and pepper to taste and add nutmeg.
4. Remove from heat and stir in cream.
5. Serve garnished with chopped hazelnuts.

W
C
Substitute yoghurt for cream if wished
Add extra stock for thinner soup
Veg

Spinach Soup

Serves 4

UK

15g/½ oz butter or margarine
1 small onion, finely sliced
225g/8 oz potatoes, peeled and diced
450g/1 lb spinach, washed and finely
    shredded
600ml/1 pint stock
salt
pepper
generous pinch nutmeg
3 tablespoons single cream

US

1¼ tablespoons butter or margarine
1 small onion, finely sliced
half pound potatoes, peeled and diced
1 pound spinach, washed and finely
    shredded
2½ cups stock
salt
pepper
generous pinch nutmeg
3 tablespoons light cream

1. Melt the butter in a large saucepan, stir in onion and potato.
2. Cover pan with lid and cook over low heat, shaking pan occasionally until vegetables are glossy.
3. Add spinach and stock, bring to boil, then simmer until potatoes are soft.
4. Blend to a purée. Season with salt and pepper and add nutmeg.
5. Reheat soup and add extra stock if necessary. Take off heat and stir in cream.

C
W
D — if vegetable margarine and
        cream are substituted
Veg

Vichyssoise

Serves 4

UK

750g/1½ lb leeks, trimmed and open
  green tops removed
750g/1½ lb potatoes, peeled
1.2 litres/2 pints chicken or vegetable
  stock
pinch ground nutmeg
150ml/¼ pint creamy milk or single
  cream
salt
pepper
1 tablespoon freshly chopped parsley

US

1½ pounds leeks, trimmed and open
  green tops removed
1½ pounds potatoes, peeled
5 cups chicken or vegetable stock
pinch ground nutmeg
⅔ cup creamy milk or light cream
salt
pepper
1 tablespoon freshly chopped parsley

1. Wash and finely slice leeks and cut potatoes into small chunks.
2. Combine in large saucepan with stock and nutmeg.
3. Simmer covered for 45 minutes or until vegetables are soft.
4. Sieve or blend, cover and leave to cool.
5. Stir in milk or cream and season to taste with salt and pepper.
6. Chill until ice cold.
7. Serve garnished with chopped parsley.

The addition of 3 or 4 ice cubes will help to chill the cooled soup more quickly.

W	
C	
D	— if soya milk substituted
Veg	— if using vegetable stock

STARTERS

Artichoke Coracles

Serves 4

UK

1 × 390g/14 oz can artichoke bottoms
175g/6 oz fromage frais
pepper
salt
1 tablespoon lumpfish caviar
box of cress

US

6-8 artichoke bottoms
⅔ cup fromage frais
pepper
salt
1 tablespoon lumpfish caviar
box of cress

1. Drain the artichoke bottoms thoroughly.
2. Season the fromage frais generously with pepper, and sparingly with salt.
3. Spoon into the artichoke bottoms.
4. Sprinkle tops with caviar.
5. Prepare the cress and spread on a serving platter and arrange the stuffed artichoke bottoms on top.

C
W
Low tyramine cheese

Artichokes Niçoise

Serves 4 to 5

UK

1 × 390g/14 oz tin artichoke hearts,
    drained and quartered
1 small onion, chopped
50g/2 oz cooked French beans, cut into
    2.5-cm/1-inch lengths
4 to 5 tablespoons French dressing [see
    page 131]
2 little gem lettuces, washed
coarsely ground black pepper
1 × 50g/1¾ oz tin anchovy fillets, well
    drained and cut in half lengthways
8 black olives

US

14 ounces canned artichoke hearts,
    drained and quartered
1 small onion, chopped
½ cup cooked French beans, cut into
    1-inch lengths
4 to 5 tablespoons French dressing [see
    page 131]
2 little gem lettuces, washed
coarsely ground black pepper
1¾ oz can anchovy fillets, well drained
    and cut in half lengthways
8 black olives

1. Put the artichoke hearts, onion and
   beans in a bowl.
2. Add dressing and toss well.
3. Line individual dishes with lettuce
   leaves.
4. Spoon mixture on to lettuce.
5. Sprinkle generously with pepper.
6. Arrange a trellis of anchovy fillets
   and olives on top.

C
W
D
Substitute gherkins if olives
unsuitable

Avocado Fans With Raspberry Coulis

Serves 4

UK

2 large ripe avocados
100g/4 oz raspberries
1–2 teaspoons maple syrup
¼ teaspoon ground nutmeg

US

2 large ripe avocados
⁴/₅ cup raspberries
1–2 teaspoons maple syrup
¼ teaspoon ground nutmeg

1. Peel the avocados, halve lengthways and remove the stones (pits).
2. Place rounded side up on a chopping board. Using a sharp stainless steel knife cut 5 vertical slices from within 2cm/¾ inch of the narrow end. Place on individual plates and press down lightly so that the slices fan out.
3. Purée and sieve the raspberries and mix with the maple syrup and nutmeg.
4. Place 1 or 2 spoonfuls of the purée on each plate beside the avocado.

C
W
D
Veg

Avocado Salad Piquant

Serves 4

UK and US

2 ripe avocados
5 tablespoons cooked mayonnaise [see
  page 128]
1 level tablespoon fresh chopped parsley
½ teaspoon fresh chopped tarragon
  leaves
4 cocktail gherkins, chopped
1 level tablespoon capers, chopped
1 radicchio lettuce, washed
12 baby tomatoes

1. Halve the avocados lengthways and
    discard the stones (pits). Spread a
    thin layer of mayonnaise over cut
    surfaces.
2. Mix parsley, tarragon, chopped
    gherkins and capers into remaining
    mayonnaise and spoon into avocado
    cavities.
3. Arrange radicchio leaves on
    individual plates. Place an avocado
    half in the centre. Halve the tomatoes
    and place cut side down on the
    radicchio leaves.

> **C**
> **D** — if non-dairy mayonnaise is
>   used
> **W**
> **Veg**

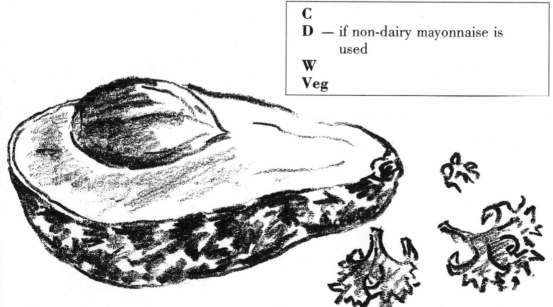

Baked Mushrooms

Serves 4 to 8

UK

8 medium open flat mushrooms
5 tablespoons hot vegetable stock
225g/8 oz cottage cheese
yolk of one hard-boiled egg, sieved
large pinch cayenne
salt
pepper
8 rounds cut from small loaf, toasted
parsley sprigs to garnish

US

8 medium open flat mushrooms
5 tablespoons hot vegetable stock
1 cup pot cheese
yolk of one hard-cooked egg, sieved
large pinch cayenne
salt
pepper
8 rounds cut from small loaf, toasted
parsley sprigs to garnish

1. Wipe mushrooms, trim and chop stalks.
2. Sprinkle with stock [this prevents mushrooms from drying out under the grill (broiler)].
3. Mix cottage (pot) cheese, chopped mushroom stalks, sieved egg yolk, cayenne and salt and pepper to taste.
4. Spread over dark side of mushrooms.
5. Grill (broil) under medium heat for 4 to 5 minutes until biscuit-coloured.
6. Place mushrooms on toasts and garnish with parsley.

Low tyramine cheese
C
Low fat
W — if toast omitted
Veg

Beetroot and Pink Prawn Salad

Serves 4

UK

4 small beetroot, cooked and peeled
1 tablespoon French dressing (see page 131)
150ml/¼ pint non-dairy single cream
75g/3 oz cooked peeled prawns
salt
freshly ground black pepper
4 cooked unshelled prawns

US

4 small beet, cooked and peeled
1 tablespoon French dressing (see page 131)
⅔ cup non-dairy light cream
½ cup cooked peeled shrimp
salt
freshly ground black pepper
4 cooked unshucked shrimp

1. Using a grapefruit knife, hollow out the beetroot (beet) leaving a thin but sturdy wall.
2. Brush with the French dressing.
3. Chop the removed centres and mix with half the peeled prawns (shrimp) and 1 tablespoon cream. Pile into the beetroot hollows [it will protrude above].
4. Finely chop the remaining peeled prawns (shrimp) and mix with the remaining cream and salt and pepper to taste.
5. When ready to serve, arrange the beetroot in the centre of individual plates and surround with the prawn (shrimp) cream.
6. Garnish each plate with a whole prawn (shrimp).

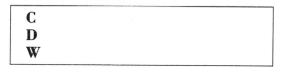

C
D
W

Dolmades

Serves 4

UK

20 to 30 large vine leaves [from a can or
    packet]
1 small onion, finely chopped
1 tablespoon olive oil
175g/6 oz brown rice, cooked
2 level teaspoons chopped mint
1 level tablespoon chopped parsley
50g/2 oz pine nuts
salt
pepper

US

20 to 30 large vine leaves [from a can or
    packet]
1 small onion, finely chopped
1 tablespoon olive oil
⅔ cup brown rice, cooked
2 level teaspoons chopped mint
1 level tablespoon chopped parsley
½ cup pine nuts
salt
pepper

C
W
D
Veg

1. Drain the vine leaves. Immerse in a
    pan of boiling water, then drain and
    refresh in cold water. Drain.
2. Fry the onion in the oil for 2
    minutes.
3. Mix into the rice with the mint,
    parsley, nuts and salt and pepper to
    taste.
4. Place a teaspoonful of filling on one
    edge of each vine leaf and roll up
    tucking in the sides.
5. Tightly pack a large frying pan
    (skillet) with the stuffed vine leaves
    seam sides down. A second layer
    may be added if separated with extra
    vine leaves.
6. Barely cover with hot water and put a
    plate greased on the underside
    directly on top of the vine leaves to
    keep them flat.
7. Cover the pan and simmer for 30 to
    40 minutes, topping up with hot
    water if necessary.
8. Remove the dolmades from the pan
    and serve warm or cold with a tomato
    and black olive salad.

Hummus

Serves 4

UK

100g/4 oz dried chick peas, soaked and
    cooked or 200g/8 oz cooked or tinned
    chick peas
2 cloves garlic
½ teaspoon salt
¼ teaspoon ground cumin
1 teaspoon paprika
¼ teaspoon freshly ground black pepper
1 tablespoon cider vinegar
3 to 4 tablespoons water
2 tomatoes, skinned, chopped and
    deseeded
100g/4 oz Tahini paste
1 small onion, finely chopped
2 level tablespoons freshly chopped
    parsley

US

½ cup dried garbanzos, soaked and
    cooked or 1 cup cooked or canned
    garbanzos
2 cloves garlic
½ teaspoon salt
¼ teaspoon ground cumin
1 teaspoon paprika
¼ teaspoon freshly ground black pepper
1 tablespoon cider vinegar
3 to 4 tablespoons water

2 tomatoes, skinned, chopped and
    deseeded
⅓ cup Tahini paste
1 small onion, finely chopped
2 level tablespoons freshly chopped
    parsley

1. Purée the chick peas (garbanzos),
    garlic, salt, cumin, paprika, pepper,
    vinegar, water and tomatoes together
    in a blender. Mix in the Tahini paste.
2. Adjust seasoning and add more
    vinegar if wished.
3. Serve with pitta bread if acceptable
    and garnish with onion and chopped
    parsley.

C
W — if served with non-wheat toast
D
Vegan

Leeks Ambala

Serves 4

UK & US

2 large leeks
4–6 tablespoons gram flour
pinch bay leaf powder
salt
freshly ground black pepper
sunflower (safflower) oil for frying

1. Trim leeks and remove green part.
2. Cut white part into approximately 2.5cm/1 inch lengths.
3. Cook in boiling water for 10 minutes or until just tender. Drain.
   OR cook without added water, but closely covered, in the microwave oven for about 5 minutes.
4. Make a thick batter with the gram flour and 2 to 4 tablespoons water.
5. Add bay leaf powder and season to taste with salt and pepper.
6. Dip the leek pieces [which should still be whole] individually into the batter, making sure that they are completely coated.
7. Heat 3 to 4 tablespoons oil in a small frying pan (skillet) and, when hot, fry the battered leeks, turning them over as soon as they are brown underneath.
8. Drain on paper towels.

Serve dry or with a tomato curry sauce [see page 133] if wished.

C
No egg
W
D
Vegan

Madras Eggs

Serves 4

UK & US

1 slice onion, chopped
1 teaspoon sunflower (safflower) oil
2 teaspoons curry powder
pinch garlic salt
½ teaspoon salt
1 tablespoon tomato purée
generous dash Worcestershire or
    Holbrooks sauce
8 tablespoons water
4 eggs, freshly hard-boiled (hard-cooked)
    and halved lengthways
1 tablespoon freshly chopped coriander

1. Gently fry the onion in the oil for 1 minute.
2. Stir in the curry powder and cook for 1 minute, stirring continuously.
3. Mix in garlic salt, salt, tomato purée, Worcestershire or Holbrooks sauce and the water. Cook for 2 to 3 minutes, stirring continuously until thickened.
4. Arrange two egg halves, curved side up, on individual plates. Coat with sauce and sprinkle with coriander.

C
W
D
Veg

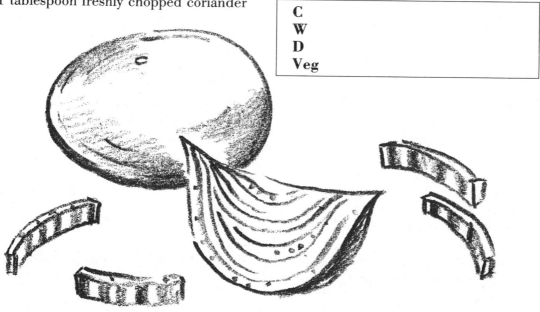

Ratatouille

Serves 4

UK

2 onions, sliced
2 cloves garlic, crushed
3–4 tablespoons sunflower oil
1 large aubergine, sliced
2 courgettes, trimmed and sliced
1 red pepper, cored, deseeded and
  sliced
1 green pepper, cored, deseeded and
  sliced
4 tomatoes, skinned and chopped
2 level tablespoons tomato purée
pinch sugar
salt
pepper
Worcestershire sauce

US

2 onions, sliced
2 cloves garlic, crushed
3–4 tablespoons safflower oil
1 large eggplant, sliced
2 zuccini, trimmed and sliced
1 red pepper, cored, deseeded and
  sliced
1 green pepper, cored, deseeded and
  sliced
4 tomatoes, skinned and chopped
2 level tablespoons tomato paste
pinch sugar

salt
pepper
Worcestershire sauce

1. Fry onion and garlic in the oil until
   soft.
2. Add aubergine (eggplant) slices a few
   at a time and fry briskly.
3. Reduce heat and add courgettes
   (zuccini), sliced peppers and
   tomatoes.
4. Cook, stirring frequently for 10
   minutes.
5. Mix in tomato purée (paste), sugar,
   salt and pepper to taste, a dash of
   Worcestershire sauce and 3 to 4
   tablespoons water.
6. Reduce heat, cover and cook gently
   for 30 to 40 minutes, checking
   occasionally to make sure vegetables
   have not dried out.
5. Adjust seasoning. Cool.

Can be served hot if wished as a vegetable.

C
W
D
Veg — if Holbrooks sauce used in place of Worcestershire

Salad Gitta

Serves 4 to 6

UK

1 small frisée lettuce
10 walnut halves
1 small ripe mango
1 red dessert apple
4 celery stalks
150ml/¼ pint natural yoghurt
salt
pepper
1 teaspoon curry powder
1 teaspoon mango chutney
4–6 slices Parma ham, cut into thin strips

US

1 small escarole lettuce
10 English walnut halves
1 small ripe mango
1 red dessert apple
4 celery stalks
⅔ cups plain yoghurt
salt
pepper
1 teaspoon curry powder
1 teaspoon mango chutney
4–6 slices Parma ham, cut into thin strips

1. Wash the lettuce, remove any tough stalk and separate the leaves.
2. Cut the leaves into bite-sized lengths and arrange on individual dishes [scallop shells show this salad off to advantage].
3. Put the walnut halves in a small saucepan, cover generously with cold water and bring to the boil. Drain in a sieve and refresh under running water. Drain thoroughly, then coarsely chop.
4. Peel and stone (pit) the mango and coarsely chop the flesh.
5. Wash, quarter, core and slice the apple. Thinly slice the celery.
6. Put the yoghurt in a large bowl, season sparingly with salt and pepper and stir in the curry powder and mango chutney.
7. Add the walnuts, mango, apple and celery and toss gently.
8. Pile the mixture on to the lettuce-lined dishes and decorate with the Parma ham.

C
W
D — if soya yoghurt or non-dairy cream substituted

MAIN DISHES

Chicken Rosemary

Serves 4

UK

2 level teaspoons chopped rosemary
    leaves
1 tablespoon sunflower oil
4 chicken breasts, skinned
salt
pepper
50g/2 oz flour

US

2 level teaspoons chopped rosemary
    leaves
1 tablespoon safflower oil
4 chicken breasts, skinned
salt
pepper
½ cup flour

1. Soak the rosemary in the oil and set aside for 30 minutes to soften.
2. Season both sides of the chicken breasts, brush with the mixture and pierce with a skewer or fork.
3. Dip the chicken in the flour and fry in a non-stick frying pan (skillet) for 8 to 10 minutes or until thoroughly cooked.

C
D
W — if fine cornmeal or gram flour substituted for flour

Chinese Egg Fried Rice

Serves 4

UK

225g/8 oz long grain rice
1 teaspoon sesame oil
1 tablespoon Tamari sauce
pinch five spice
freshly ground black pepper
90g/3½ oz tin tuna in brine, drained and
  flaked
50g/2 oz beansprouts, rinsed and
  drained
2 eggs, beaten

US

1 cup long grain rice
1 teaspoon sesame oil
1 tablespoon Tamari sauce
pinch five spice
freshly ground black pepper
3½ oz can tuna in brine, drained and
  flaked
1 cup beansprouts, rinsed and drained
2 eggs, beaten

1. Boil the rice in your usual way and immediately stir the sesame seed oil, Tamari, five spice and a generous shake of black pepper into the freshly cooked hot rice.
2. Mix in the tuna and beansprouts. Cover the saucepan and keep warm.
3. Pour the eggs into a lightly oiled frying pan (skillet) and cook until set.
4. Turn the omelette over to brown the other side.
5. Remove from the pan, roll up Swiss roll (jelly roll) fashion, then cut into very thin strips.
6. Stir into the rice mixture and serve immediately.

Suitable for vegetarians if diced firm tofu is substituted for tuna.

W
MSG
C
D

Crumble-Baked Chicken

Serves 4

UK

120g/4 oz brown rice flour
25g/1 oz arrowroot
60g/2 oz ground almonds
2 level teaspoons dried sage
1 tablespoon freshly chopped parsley
½ teaspoon salt
¼ teaspoon pepper
3 tablespoons olive oil
4 chicken breasts or drumsticks, skinned
2 eggs, beaten

US

¾ cup brown rice flour
1 oz arrowroot
½ cup ground almonds
2 level teaspoons dried sage
1 tablespoon freshly chopped parsley
½ teaspoon salt
¼ teaspoon pepper
3 tablespoons olive oil
4 chicken breasts or drumsticks, skinned
2 eggs, beaten

1. Thoroughly mix the dry ingredients together.
2. Sprinkle with the oil and fork through. [Do not overmix or the mixture will be too lumpy.]
3. Dip the chicken pieces in the egg and then into the crumble mix, pressing it well in and making sure all sides are evenly coated.
4. Arrange them in a single layer in a baking dish and refrigerate for 30 to 45 minutes.
5. Bake at 200°C/400°F/Gas mark 6 for 30–45 minutes until golden brown and the chicken is thoroughly cooked.

Serve with gravy or mushroom sauce [see page 121]

For special occasions make a slit in the chicken breasts and fill with paté before dipping and coating.

W
D
C

Delicious Baked Chicken

Serves 4

UK

4 chicken quarters
salt
pepper
50g/2 oz butter or magarine
75g/3 oz flaked almonds
100g/4 oz mushrooms, trimmed and
    sliced
25g/1 oz flour
50g/2 oz sultanas
250ml/8 fl oz grape juice
200ml/7 fl oz evaporated milk

US

4 chicken quarters
salt
pepper
¼ cup butter or margarine
¾ cup slivered almonds
1 cup mushrooms, trimmed and sliced
¼ cup flour
⅓ cup golden seedless raisins
1 cup grape juice
¾ cup evaporated milk

1. Heat the oven to 200°C/400°F/Gas mark 6.
2. Season the chicken with salt and pepper and place in a roasting dish. Bake for 35 to 45 minutes or until tender, turning the pieces over twice during cooking. Drain and keep hot.
3. While the chicken is baking, melt half the butter in a large pan and lightly fry the almonds. Add the mushrooms and cook for 2 minutes.
4. Add remaining butter and stir in the flour. Mix in the sultanas (raisins) and grape juice and cook until thickened.
5. Stir in the milk and cook gently for a further 10 minutes.

Serve the chicken topped with the sauce and accompanied by mashed potatoes or rice.

C
W — if substitute 1 tablespoon potato flour for wheat flour, first mixing with a little of the grape juice
D — if vegetable margarine and milk are substituted

Devilled Mushrooms

Serves 4 as a main course or 6 as a starter

UK

450g/1 lb button mushrooms
25g/1 oz butter
2 teaspoons tomato purée
1 teaspoon Worcestershire or Holbrooks
  sauce
1 teaspoon French mustard
½ teaspoon sugar
salt
freshly ground black pepper
4 tablespoons single cream

US

4 cups button mushrooms
2½ tablespoons butter
2 teaspoons tomato paste
1 teaspoon Worcestershire or Holbrooks
  sauce
1 teaspoon French mustard
½ teaspoon sugar
salt
freshly ground black pepper
4 tablespoons light cream

1. Wipe the mushrooms.
2. Melt the butter in a large frying pan (skillet) and sauté the mushrooms for 5 to 6 minutes until tender.
3. Remove mushrooms from pan and stir tomato purée (paste), sauce, mustard and sugar into juices. Cook for 2 to 4 minutes until reduced to a creamy pouring consistency. Season to taste with salt and pepper.
4. Stir the mushrooms into the sauce, cover and cook until they are hot. Stir in the cream and remove the pan from the heat.

Serve hot on croûtes of fried or toasted bread or with rice or in nests of mashed potato. Can also be served cold with an egg and watercress salad.

C
W
D — if non-dairy cream substituted
Veg — and vegans if non-dairy cream and Holbrooks sauce are used

Grilled Plaice, Japanese Style

Serves 4

UK

6 tablespoons Miso
1 tablespoon demerara sugar
3 tablespoons grape juice
25g/1 oz vegetable margarine
3 large plaice, heads removed, cleaned
and gutted
4–5 spring onions, trimmed and thinly
sliced diagonally

US

6 tablespoons Miso
1 tablespoon demerara sugar
3 tablespoons grape juice
2½ tablespoons vegetable margarine
3 large plaice, heads removed, cleaned
and cutted
4–5 scallions, trimmed and thinly sliced
diagonally

1. Combine the Miso, sugar and grape juice in a small saucepan.
2. Cook over gentle heat, stirring continuously until thick.
3. Stir in margarine and remove from heat.
4. Cut fish in half lengthways and, using a sharp knife, loosen flesh from either side of bone to form a pocket.
5. Brush with sauce on both the inside and outside of the fish.
6. Grill (broil) fish under a medium grill for 4 to 5 minutes on each side until cooked, then brush with any remaining sauce.
7. Serve hot garnished with spring onions (scallions).

W
C
D — but substitute butter if wished

Grilled Salmon With Dill Sauce

Serves 4

UK

4×175g/6 oz salmon steaks
salt
pepper
50g/2 oz butter
Dill weed sauce [see page 129]

US

4×175g/6 oz salmon steaks
salt
pepper
¼ cup butter
Dill weed sauce [see page 129]

1. Rinse salmon steaks and pat dry on paper towel.
2. Season with salt and pepper and top with dabs of butter.
3. Preheat medium grill (broiler) and cook the salmon for 10 to 12 minutes [there should be no need to turn the fish over].
4. Spoon sauce over hot salmon and serve as it melts.

Serve with steamed new potatoes.

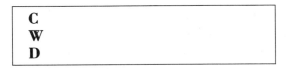

C
W
D

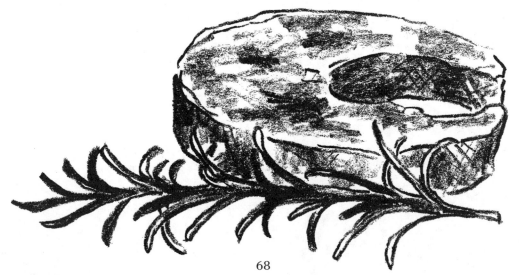

Grilled Trout Veronique

Serves 4

UK & US

225g/8 oz green grapes
6 tablespoons unsweetened apple juice
1 tablespoon sunflower (safflower) oil
1 level teaspoon chopped mint
salt
freshly ground black pepper
4 trout, gutted and cleaned

1. Skin and de-pip the grapes. Set aside 12 grapes for garnish and chop remainder.
2. Mix chopped grapes, apple juice, oil and mint and season to taste with salt and pepper.
3. Score through fish with a sharp knife at about 2.5cm/1 inch intervals.
4. Fill open flaps underneath the fish with grape mixture. Arrange in a single layer in a shallow dish and pour remaining mixture over.
5. Cover and refrigerate for about 30 minutes.
6. Preheat a medium grill (broiler) and cook fish on the rack for 7 to 8 minutes on each side.
7. Meanwhile reheat the grape marinade and reserved grapes.
8. Pour hot mixture over trout and serve hot.

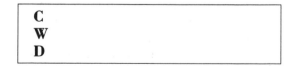

C
W
D

Haddock and Avocado Tartines

Serves 4

UK & US

4×100–175g/4–6 oz cutlets fresh
  haddock or similar white fish
7 tablespoons milk
7 tablespoons water
1 tablespoon chopped chives
1 bay leaf
1 blade mace
3 tablespoons quick cook porridge oats
½ teaspoon lemon thyme
1 egg, beaten
salt
pepper
1 ripe avocado
paprika

1. Rinse fish and pat dry with paper towel.
2. Combine milk, water, chives, bay leaf and mace in a large frying pan (skillet).
3. Bring to simmering point, place the fish cutlets in a single layer in the pan, cover and reduce heat. Poach gently for 8 to 10 minutes until fish is white and flaky.
4. Remove skin and bones, bay leaf and mace.
5. Stir oats into 5 tablespoons of the fish liquid, making up with more milk if necessary. Add lemon thyme. Heat for 1 minute then leave to cool for 10 minutes. Mix in beaten egg and add seasoning.
6. Meanwhile grease 4×150ml/5 fl oz/⅔ cup individual tartlet tins or ramekins. Flake the fish.
7. Press a layer of fish into each mould, cover with the oat mixture and finish with a layer of fish. Press down with a fork.
8. Cover tartlet tins tightly with greased foil, place in large baking tin and pour about 2.5cm/1 inch hot water into the tin. Bake at 180°C/350°F/Gas mark 4 for 45 minutes to 1 hour.
9. Remove tartlet tins from oven and leave to cool. Refrigerate.
10. Just before serving, mash the avocado, smooth over fish and garnish with a shake of paprika.

Serve cold with salad.

If preferred the tartines may be unmoulded with aid of a grapefruit knife before coating with the avocado.

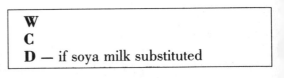

W
C
D — if soya milk substituted

Herrings in Oatmeal

Serves 4

UK

4 herrings
salt
pepper
50–75g/2–3 oz coarse oatmeal
25g/1 oz butter or margarine

US

4 herrings
salt
pepper
⅔ cup coarse oatmeal
2½ tablespoons butter or margarine

1. Remove the heads, slit along the underside and clean and rinse the fish thoroughly.
2. To remove bones, open out underside with the fingers and place on paper towel, skin side up. Press all along the back bone which will loosen the bones, then reverse fish and lift bone from flesh.
3. Season the fish on the open side. Reshape the fish and coat thoroughly in oatmeal, pressing in with a palette knife.
4. Melt butter in a large non-stick frying pan (skillet) and fry the fish over medium heat for 3 to 4 minutes on each side.

C
W
D — if vegetable margarine substituted

Hungarian Goulyas

Serves 4 to 6

UK

3-4 tablespoons single cream
½ teaspoon malt vinegar
2 medium onions, chopped
1 clove garlic, crushed
1 green pepper, cored, seeded and cut
    into strips
2-3 tablespoons salad oil
1kg/2 lb lean braising steak, cut into
    2.5-cm/1-inch pieces.
2 tablespoons sweet paprika
2 tablespoons tomato purée
2 tablespoons cornflour
4 tomatoes, skinned and quartered
450ml/¾ pint stock or water
salt
freshly ground black pepper

US

3-4 tablespoons light cream
½ teaspoon malt vinegar
2 medium onions, chopped
1 clove garlic, crushed
1 green pepper, cored, seeded and cut
    into strips
2—3 tablespoons salad oil
2 pounds lean braising steak, cut into
    1-inch pieces.
2 tablespoons sweet paprika
2 tablespoons tomato paste
2 tablespoons cornstarch
4 tomatoes, skinned and quartered
2 cups stock or water
salt
freshly ground black pepper

1. Blend cream and vinegar together
   and leave for 30 minutes.
2. Fry onions, garlic and pepper in the
   oil for 3 to 4 minutes until tender.
3. Add meat cubes a few at a time and
   fry briskly until browned on all sides.
4. Add paprika, tomato purée (paste)
   and cornflour (cornstarch) blended
   together with 2 tablespoons water.
5. Cook, stirring for 2 minutes.
6. Add tomatoes, stock and salt and
   pepper to taste.
7. Cover and simmer for 2 to 2½ hours
   until meat is tender.
8. Just before serving, stir in blended
   cream and vinegar.

C
W
No wine
D — if non-dairy cream substituted

Kichkiri

Serves 4

UK

1 tablespoon sunflower oil
1 medium onion, finely chopped
1 garlic clove, crushed
¼ teaspoon turmeric
¼ teaspoon ground cinnamon
pinch ground cloves
2 pods cardamom, cracked
75g/3 oz long grain rice
75g/3 oz red lentils
450ml/¾ pint hot water
salt
pepper
3 tablespoons natural yoghurt
2 eggs, hard-boiled, sliced

US

1 tablespoon safflower oil
1 medium onion, finely chopped,
1 garlic clove, crushed
¼ teaspoon turmeric
¼ teaspoon ground cinnamon
pinch ground cloves
2 pods cardamom, cracked
½ cup long grain rice
⅔ cup red lentils
2 cups hot water
salt
pepper

3 tablespoons plain yoghurt
2 eggs, hard-cooked, sliced

1. Combine oil, onion, garlic and spices
   in a large saucepan. Cover and cook
   5 minutes until onion is tender.
2. Stir in rice, lentils and hot water.
   Bring to the boil, then lower heat and
   simmer covered for 20 minutes,
   stirring occasionally to prevent
   sticking until lentils are cooked and
   most of the liquid is absorbed.
   Remove pan from heat and leave
   covered for 10 minutes.
3. Season with salt and pepper. Stir in
   yoghurt.
4. Spoon mixture into warm serving
   dish and garnish with egg slices.

Vegans may wish to omit egg and
substitute toasted nuts.

W
C
D — if non-dairy cream substituted
Veg

Lamb and Pine Nut Patties

Serves 4 to 6

UK

1kg/2 lb minced lean leg of lamb
1 small onion, very finely chopped
½ teaspoon ground nutmeg
salt
freshly ground black pepper
75g/3 oz pine nuts, chopped
2 tablespoons vegetable oil

US

4 cups ground lean leg of lamb
1 small onion, very finely chopped
½ teaspoon ground nutmeg
salt
freshly ground black pepper
¾ cup pine nuts, chopped
2 tablespoons vegetable oil

1. Thoroughly mix together the lamb, onion, nutmeg and season to taste with salt and pepper.
2. Mix in the pine nuts. The mixture should bind without the need to add any egg.
3. Divide into 12 balls and flatten to 0.5cm/½ inch thick.
4. Place on a tray and chill for 30 minutes.
5. Brush patties on both sides with oil and fry in an ungreased frying pan (skillet) over medium heat for about 8 to 10 minutes on each side.

Serve with a green salad and goat's milk feta cheese if wished.

W
C
D

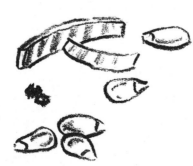
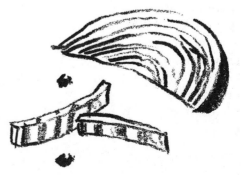

Lamb Cutlets in Cider Pepper Sauce

Serves 4 to 6

UK

8 spring onions, trimmed and finely
   sliced
1 red pepper, cored, deseeded and finely
   chopped
1 tablespoon sunflower oil
2 tablespoons cornflour
2 shakes Tabasco
200ml/7 fl oz sweet cider
salt
pepper
8 lamb cutlets, trimmed of all fat

US

8 scallions, trimmed and finely sliced
1 red pepper, cored, deseeded and finely
   chopped
1 tablespoon safflower oil
2 tablespoons cornstarch
2 shakes Tabasco
⅔ cup sweet cider
salt
pepper
8 lamb cutlets, trimmed of all fat

1. Fry spring onions (scallions) and red pepper in the oil until soft.
2. Blend cornflour (cornstarch), Tabasco and cider.
3. Pour into pan of spring onions (scallions) and peppers. Bring to boil, stirring continuously until sauce thickens.
4. Season to taste with salt and pepper and keep hot.
5. Grill (broil) cutlets under medium heat for 4 to 5 minutes on each side.
6. Serve cutlets with sauce.

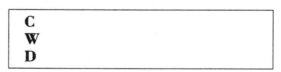

C
W
D

Moussaka

Serves 4 to 5

UK

1 aubergine, peeled and thinly sliced
4 to 6 tablespoons sunflower oil
1 onion, finely chopped
½ clove garlic, crushed
225g/8 oz potato, peeled and sliced
   lengthways
350g/12 oz lamb or beef
2 tomatoes, skinned and chopped
2 tablespoons tomato purée
¼ teaspoon cinnamon
salt, pepper
1 egg yolk
450ml/¾ pint Béchamel sauce [see page
   120]

US

1 eggplant, peeled and thinly sliced
4 to 6 tablespoons safflower oil
1 onion, finely chopped
½ clove garlic, crushed
1 cup potato, peeled and sliced
   lengthways
1½ cups lamb or beef
2 tomatoes, skinned and chopped
2 tablespoons tomato paste
¼ teaspoon cinnamon
salt, pepper
1 egg yolk
2 cups Béchamel sauce [see page 120]

1. Spread aubergine (eggplant) slices in colander over a bowl. Sprinkle with salt. Leave 30 minutes. Drain, rinse and pat dry on paper towel.
2. Heat 2 to 3 tablespoons oil in large non-stick frying pan (skillet) and fry onion, garlic and aubergine (eggplant) slices. Remove and drain on paper towel. Add more oil to pan and gently fry sliced potato. Remove from pan.
3. Without adding more oil, fry meat, stirring briskly until browned.
4. Stir in tomatoes, tomato purée (paste), cinnamon and add salt sparingly.
5. Add pepper and 2–3 tablespoons water. Simmer for 15 minutes.
6. Arrange layers of aubergine (eggplant), meat and potatoes in deep oven-proof dish. Beat egg yolk into Béchamel sauce and pour over top.
7. Bake at 190°C/375°F/Gas mark 5 for 45 minutes or until brown on top.

No cheese
C
D   — if soya milk is substituted
         when making sauce
Omit egg yolk for lower cholesterol
Veg — if substitute cooked kidney
         beans for meat

Smoky Tofu Stir-fry

Serves 4 to 5

UK

225g/8 oz block smoked tofu
2 tablespoons Tamari
2 tablespoons dry sherry
5 tablespoons cold water
1 tablespoon cornflour
3 tablespoons sunflower oil
75g/3 oz beansprouts
50g/2 oz green beans, sliced diagonally
4–6 spring onions, trimmed and sliced
small red pepper, cored, seeded and cut
   into rings
4 water chestnuts, sliced
75g/3 oz sweetcorn kernels
1 garlic clove, crushed
2 teaspoons very finely chopped ginger
   root
Freshly cooked rice or noodles

US

8 ounce block smoked tofu
2 tablespoons Tamari
2 tablespoons dry sherry
5 tablespoons cold water
1 tablespoon cornstarch
3 tablespoons safflower oil
1½ cups beansprouts
½ cup green beans, sliced diagonally
4–6 scallions, trimmed and sliced
small red pepper, cored, seeded and cut
   into rings
4 water chestnuts, sliced
½ cup sweetcorn kernels
1 garlic clove, crushed
2 teaspoons very finely chopped ginger
   root
Freshly cooked rice or noodles

1. Cut the tofu into
   5cm × 5mm × 5mm/2 inch × ¼
   inch × ¼ inch strips and pat dry on
   paper towel.
2. Blend the Tamari, sherry, water and
   cornflour (cornstarch) until smooth.
3. Heat the oil in a wok or large frying
   pan (skillet) and fry the strips a few
   at a time until brown. Drain on paper
   towel.
4. Add a little more oil to wok if
   necessary, heat briskly and stir-fry
   the vegetables, garlic and ginger for
   2 to 3 minutes.
5. Add the blended sauce and stir until
   thickened. Quickly mix in the tofu
   strips to reheat.
6. Serve at once on bed of rice or
   noodles.

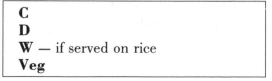

C
D
W — if served on rice
Veg

Somerset Beef and Walnut Pie

Serves 4 to 5

UK

1 tablespoon sunflower oil
1 onion, chopped
1 baby turnip, peeled and sliced
350g/12 oz freshly minced beef
4–5 pickled walnuts, sliced
1 tablespoon tomato purée
2 tomatoes, quartered
1 dessert apple, cored, peeled and
    chopped
salt
freshly ground black pepper
350g/12 oz mashed potato

US

1 tablespoon safflower oil
1 onion, chopped
1 baby turnip, peeled and diced
1½ cups freshly ground beef
4–5 pickled English walnuts, sliced
1 tablespoon tomato paste
2 tomatoes quartered
1 dessert apple, cored, peeled and
    chopped
salt
freshly ground black pepper
1½ cups mashed potato

1. Heat the oil and fry the onion for 3 to 4 minutes until soft.
2. Add turnip and fry gently for 5 minutes.
3. Raise heat and fry meat briskly a little at a time to brown on all sides.
4. Mix in walnuts, tomato purée (paste), tomatoes, apple and season to taste with salt and pepper.
5. Pour into an oven-proof dish. Top with potato and fork up the surface.
6. Bake in a pre-heated oven 180°C/350°F/Gas mark 4 for 40 to 50 minutes.

C
W
D

Spinach Soufflé

Serves 4 to 5

UK

40g/1½ oz butter or margarine
2 tablespoons cornflour
225ml/8 fl oz milk
½ teaspoon salt
¼ teaspoon freshly ground black pepper
225g/8 oz cooked spinach, very finely
    chopped [chopped frozen spinach can
    be used]
generous shake ground nutmeg
4 egg yolks, beaten
5 egg whites

US

3 tablespoons butter or margarine
2 tablespoons cornstarch
1 cup milk
⅓ teaspoon salt
¼ teaspoon freshly ground black pepper
2 cups cooked spinach, very finely
    chopped [chopped frozen spinach can
    be used]
generous shake ground nutmeg
4 egg yolks, beaten
5 egg whites

1. Grease a 1.5 litre/2½ pint/6½ cup soufflé dish well.
2. Melt butter or margarine in medium saucepan. Remove from heat and stir in cornflour (cornstarch). Gradually blend in milk.
3. Cook over low heat, stirring continuously, until sauce boils and thickens. Season with salt and pepper.
4. Remove from heat. Stir in spinach and nutmeg to taste.
5. Leave for 15 to 20 minutes to cool. Stir in beaten egg yolks.
6. Heat oven to 180°C/350°F/Gas mark 4.
7. Whisk egg whites to soft peaks in grease-free bowl. Stir 1 tablespoon whisked egg whites into spinach sauce.
8. Fold in remainder of egg whites with large metal spoon.
9. Pour mixture into prepared soufflé dish and place in large baking tin, containing 2.5cm/1 inch hot water.
10. Bake for about 1 hour until puffed up and no longer runny inside.

No cheese
W
C
D — if soya milk and vegetable
        margarine substituted
Veg

Summer Peach Chicken

Serves 4 to 6

UK

1 × 1.5kg/3½ lb roasted chicken, cold
salt
pepper
4 spring onions, trimmed and chopped
1 red pepper, cored, deseeded and
    sliced into rings
6 slender sticks celery
150ml/¼ pint mayonnaise [see page
    128]
2 fresh peaches, skinned and sliced
watercress

US

1 × 3½ pound roasted chicken, cold
salt
pepper
4 scallions, trimmed and chopped
1 red pepper, cored, deseeded and
    sliced into rings
6 centre sticks celery
⅔ cup mayonnaise [see page 128]
2 fresh peaches, skinned and sliced
watercress

1. Remove skin and bones from chicken [save if wished to make chicken stock].
2. Season chicken and cut into equally sized pieces.
3. Mix with spring onions (scallions), red pepper and celery.
4. Spoon on to a large platter or individual plates.
5. Coat with mayonnaise and garnish with peach slices lightly brushed with mayonnaise to prevent discoloration.
6. Serve with watercress.

C
W
D

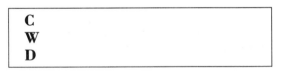

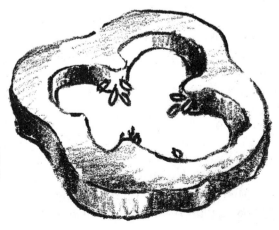

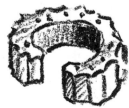

Turkey, Ham and Melon Salad

Serves 4

UK

2 small Galia melons
175g/6 oz cooked turkey
175g/6 oz ham
4–5 tablespoons mayonnaise [see page 128]
generous pinch ground ginger
1 large green pepper, cored, deseeded and cut into thin strips
4 sprigs parsley to garnish

US

2 small Galia melons
⅔ cup cooked turkey
⅔ cup ham
4–5 tablespoons mayonnaise [see page 128]
generous pinch ground ginger
1 large green pepper, cored, deseeded and cut into thin strips
4 sprigs parsley to garnish

1. Halve the melons crossways and remove the seeds. To ensure that they will stand firmly, remove a sliver from the peel on the curved side.
2. Using a baller or teaspoon, scoop out as many 'balls' as possible. Scoop out and coarsely chop the remaining flesh.
3. Cut the turkey into chunks and dice the ham.
4. Mix the mayonnaise and ginger together in a large bowl.
5. Add the ham, turkey, chopped and balled melon and toss gently to coat.
6. Fill the melon shells with the mixture and decorate with the pepper strips and parsley.

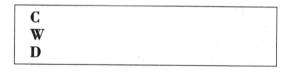

C
W
D

VEGETABLES AND SALADS

Vegetable and Nut Pilau

Serves 6 as a main course

UK

75g/3 oz vegetable margarine
350g/12 oz long grain rice, rinsed and
  drained
25g/1 oz shelled hazelnuts, finely
  chopped
25g/1 oz pine nuts
25g/1 oz cashew nuts, coarsely chopped
900ml/1½ pints well-flavoured vegetable
  stock
½ to 1 teaspoon salt
1 teaspoon ground cardamom
1 teaspoon turmeric
50g/2 oz sultanas
½ red pepper, diced
½ green pepper, diced
4 tablespoons cooked or frozen peas

US

½ cup vegetable margarine
2 cups long grain rice, rinsed and
  drained
3 tablespoons shelled hazelnuts, finely
  chopped

3 tablespoons pine nuts
3 tablespoons cashew nuts, coarsely
  chopped
3⅔ cups well-flavored vegetable stock
½ to 1 teaspoon salt
1 teaspoon ground cardamom
1 teaspoon turmeric
¼ cup golden seedless raisins
½ red pepper, diced
½ green pepper, diced
4 tablespoons cooked or frozen peas

1. Melt the margarine in a large heavy-based saucepan and stir in rice and nuts.
2. Cook, stirring continuously for about 3 minutes, until rice and nuts have a golden glow.
3. Add all remaining ingredients, stir and bring to the boil. Reduce heat, tightly cover and cook gently for 15 minutes [do not remove lid during this time].
4. Test and if rice is not yet cooked but the liquid has evaporated, add a little water or stock. If rice is cooked and liquid remains, boil without covering to evaporate excess moisture.
5. Serve hot or cold [freezes well].

W
D
C
Veg — but fish, chicken or meat   may be added.

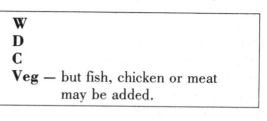

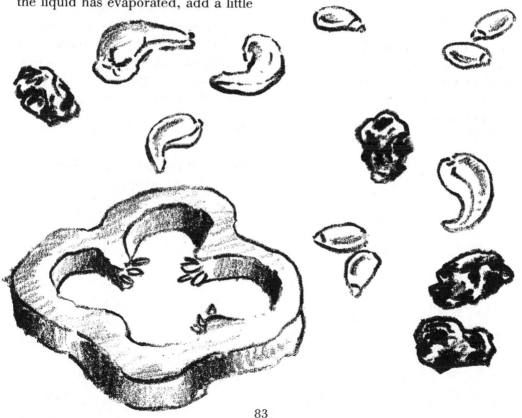

Caribbean Sweet Potatoes

Serves 6

UK

900g/2 lb sweet potatoes
50g/2 oz demerara sugar
½ teaspoon ground cinnamon
½ teaspoon ground nutmeg
150ml/¼ pint apple juice
50g/2 oz butter

US

2 pounds sweet potatoes
¼ cup demerara sugar
½ teaspoon ground cinnamon
½ teaspoon ground nutmeg
⅔ cup apple juice
¼ cup butter

1. Peel and thinly slice the potatoes.
2. Mix the sugar, cinnamon and nutmeg with the apple juice.
3. Layer the potatoes, spiced apple juice and dabs of butter in a deep baking dish, finishing with butter.
4. Cover tightly with a lid or foil.
5. Bake at 200°C/400°F/Gas mark 6 for 1 to 1½ hours, basting occasionally until the potatoes are tender and coated in a thick syrup. Add extra apple juice if the syrup becomes too thick.

Serve hot with grilled lamb or pork.

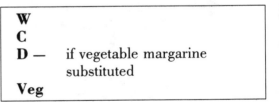

W
C
D — if vegetable margarine substituted
Veg

Carrot and Swede Purée

Serves 2 to 3

UK

1 small swede [about 285g/10 oz],
    peeled and thinly sliced
salt
350g/¾ lb carrots, peeled and sliced
pinch sugar
20g/¾ oz butter
freshly ground black pepper

US

1 small swede [about 10 ounces], peeled
    and thinly sliced
salt
1½ cups carrots, peeled and sliced
pinch sugar
2 tablespoons butter
freshly ground black pepper

1. Put swede in saucepan and cover with about 2.5cm/1 inch salted water. Cover with a lid and simmer for 15 minutes. Add the carrots and extra boiling water if necessary. Simmer covered for 15 minutes.
2. Remove lid and cook until water is almost evaporated and vegetables are tender.
3. Purée with sugar and butter. Season to taste with pepper and salt if needed.
4. Serve hot.

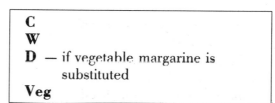

C
W
D — if vegetable margarine is
      substituted
Veg

Continental Cabbage

Serves 4

UK

1 medium-size tight-leaved cabbage
2 onions, sliced
1 garlic clove, crushed
1 tablespoon sunflower oil
2 tomatoes, skinned and sliced
2 teaspoons cornflour
300ml/½ pint stock
½ teaspoon caraway seeds
salt
pepper

US

1 medium-size tight-leaved cabbage
2 onions, sliced
1 garlic clove, crushed
1 tablespoon safflower oil
2 tomatoes, skinned and sliced
2 teaspoons cornstarch
1¼ cups stock
½ teaspoon caraway seeds
salt
pepper

1. Wash the cabbage and cut into quarters. Remove the tough central stalk.
2. Half fill a large saucepan with water, bring to the boil, add the cabbage and cook for 4 minutes. Drain.
3. Gently fry the onions and garlic in the oil until soft but not coloured.
4. Add the tomatoes and cook for 1 minute.
5. Blend the cornflour (cornstarch) and cold stock, pour into the pan, adding the caraway seeds and salt and pepper to taste.
6. Bring to the boil, stirring continuously.
7. Arrange cabbage quarters in a casserole and pour sauce over.
8. Cover and bake at 180°C/350°F/ Gas mark 4 for 45 minutes to 1 hour.

C
W
D
Low fat

Eggplant from Albuquerque

Serves 4

UK

4 medium aubergine
3 tablespoons olive oil
1 garlic clove, crushed
2 celery stalks, finely sliced
1 small onion, chopped
1 medium carrot, grated
¼ to ½ teaspoon chilli powder
1 teaspoon oregano
6 stuffed olives, sliced
1 tablespoon potato flour
1 × 225g/8 oz tin tomatoes
salt
pepper

US

4 medium eggplant
3 tablespoons olive oil
1 garlic clove, minced
2 celery stalks, finely sliced
1 small onion, chopped
1 medium carrot, grated
¼ to ½ teaspoon chilli powder
1 teaspoon oregano
6 stuffed olives, sliced
1 tablespoon potato flour
8 ounces canned tomatoes
salt
pepper

1. Remove a thin slice lengthways from one side of each aubergine (eggplant). Place aubergines in large saucepan and add water to cover. Place lid on pan and simmer for 25 minutes until flesh is tender. Remove from pan and drain.
2. Scoop out pulp with a grapefruit knife, leaving the shells intact. Cut flesh into cubes.
3. Heat oil in a large frying pan (skillet) and fry the garlic, celery and onion until tender. Add carrot, then cover and cook for 3 to 4 minutes.
4. Remove pan from heat and stir in remaining ingredients and cubed aubergine and season with salt and pepper.
5. Pile mixture into reserved aubergine (eggplant) shells.
6. Place aubergines in a single layer in a well-greased oven-proof dish.
7. Bake in a preheated oven 200°C/400°F/Gas mark 6 for 20 to 25 minutes.

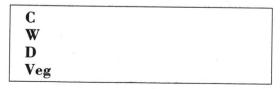

C
W
D
Veg

Golden Hash Browns

Serves 4 to 5

UK

450g/1 lb potatoes
1 small onion, very finely chopped
1 teaspoon salt
¼ teaspoon pepper
25g/1 oz butter
2 tablespoons olive oil

US

1 pound potatoes
1 small onion, very finely chopped
1 teaspoon salt
¼ teaspoon pepper
2½ tablespoons butter
2 tablespoons olive oil

1. Peel and coarsely grate the potatoes and thoroughly mix with the onion, salt and pepper.
2. Heat the butter and 1 tablespoon oil in a 23cm/9 inch frying pan (skillet) and, when foaming, add the potatoes and pack them down firmly, leaving a border around the edges.
3. Reduce heat and fry gently for 10 to 15 minutes until golden underneath.
4. Pour remaining tablespoon oil into pan and carefully turn potato cake over. Cook for 15 to 20 minutes until cooked through and browned underneath.

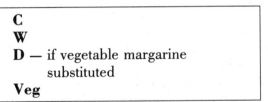

C
W
D — if vegetable margarine
     substituted
Veg

Hot 'N' Crisp Salad

Serves 4

UK

450 to 750g/1 to 1½ lb cabbage,
    trimmed, washed, thick stalks removed
3 carrots
25g/1 oz butter
8–10 chives, finely chopped
salt
pepper

US

1 to 1½ pound cabbage, trimmed,
    washed, thick stalks removed
3 carrots
2½ tablespoons butter
8–10 chives, chopped
salt
pepper

1. Shred the cabbage and scrape and grate the carrots.
2. In a large frying pan (skillet), melt the butter, add and gently cook the chives for 1 minute.
3. Stir in prepared vegetables, cover and cook over high heat, shaking the pan vigorously until tender but crisp, about 4 minutes.
4. Season to taste with salt and pepper.
5. Serve hot.

C
W
D — if vegetable margarine
    substituted
Veg

Lentil and Carrot Salad

Serves 4 to 6

UK

225g/8 oz carrots, scraped and cut into
  matchsticks
1 medium-size leek, trimmed, washed
  and thinly sliced
3 tablespoons olive oil
1 tablespoon malt vinegar
salt
freshly ground black pepper
pinch sugar
1 handful parsley sprigs, chopped
75g/3 oz green lentils, cooked

US

½ lb carrots, scraped and cut into
  matchsticks
1 medium-size leek, trimmed, washed
  and thinly sliced
3 tablespoons olive oil
1 tablespoon malt vinegar
salt
freshly ground black pepper
pinch sugar
1 handful parsley sprigs, chopped
½ cup green lentils, cooked

1. Put the carrots and leeks in large pan of boiling salted water and cook for 3 minutes.
2. Drain, reserving liquid. Cool vegetables rapidly in colander under cold running water. Drain again.
3. Combine 6 tablespoons of the cooking liquid, the oil, vinegar, salt and pepper to taste and the sugar.
4. Stir in most of the parsley.
5. Mix thoroughly with the cooked lentils. Fold in carrots and leeks.
6. Serve sprinkled with the remaining parsley.

This salad can also be served heated as a vegetable dish.

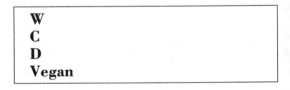

W
C
D
Vegan

Low-fat Crunchy Spinach Compôte

Serves 4

UK

500g/1¼ lb spinach, washed and thick
 stalks removed
¼ teaspoon ground coriander
freshly ground black pepper
2 tablespoons water
6 rashers lean bacon, trimmed of all fat
4 thin slices wholemeal bread, cut from a
 sandwich loaf
2 tablespoons flaked almonds

US

1¼ pounds spinach, washed and thick
 stalks removed
¼ teaspoon ground coriander
freshly ground black pepper
6 rashers lean bacon, trimmed of all fat
4 thin slices wheatmeal bread, cut from a
 sandwich loaf
2 tablespoons slivered almonds

1. Cook the spinach, adding the
   coriander and a generous shake of
   pepper in the water in a large
   covered saucepan for 8 to 10
   minutes until tender. Drain, coarsely
   chop, then return to saucepan away
   from the heat and replace lid to keep
   hot.
2. Grill (broil) the bacon until crisp. Cut
   into slivers with kitchen scissors.
3. Meanwhile remove crusts and dice
   the bread.
4. Remove the rack and spread the
   diced bread in the grill pan (broiler
   pan).
5. Toss so that the bread absorbs any
   bacon drippings and toast crisply.
6. Remove the toasted diced bread and
   lightly toast the almonds.
7. Mix the spinach with the bacon,
   almonds and toasted diced bread.
8. Spoon into a warm serving dish and
   serve immediately.

C	
D	
W	— omit bread and increase almonds
Veg	— if bacon omitted and smoked grilled tofu substituted

Pan-casseroled Corn

Serves 4 to 5

UK

4 rashers lean bacon, trimmed and diced
1 small onion, finely chopped
1 medium green pepper, cored, seeded
  and diced
450g/1 lb sweetcorn kernels
salt
pepper
3 tomatoes, skinned and chopped
1 to 2 teaspoons water
1 bay leaf

US

4 rashers lean bacon, trimmed and diced
1 small onion, finely chopped
1 medium green pepper, cored, seeded
  and diced
2⅔ cups sweetcorn kernels
salt
pepper
3 tomatoes, skinned and chopped
1 to 2 teaspoons water
1 bay leaf

1. Put bacon in large frying pan (skillet)
   and cook over low heat until fat
   oozes.
2. Add onion and green pepper and
   cook for 2–3 minutes, stirring
   continuously.
3. Stir in corn and season with salt and
   pepper.
4. Cover and cook over low heat for 15
   minutes. Stir in tomatoes and water.
   Add bay leaf, cover and continue
   cooking for 10 minutes until
   tomatoes are tender. Add salt and
   pepper if wished and remove bay
   leaf.
5. Serve hot.

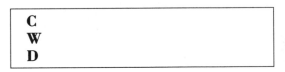

C
W
D

Potato and Chive Flan

Serves 4

UK

1kg/2 lb large potatoes
50g/2 oz butter, melted
4 tablespoons cornflour
salt
pepper
4 tablespoons double cream
¼ teaspoon white vinegar
12 chives, chopped

US

2 pounds large potatoes
¼ cup butter, melted
4 tablespoons cornstarch
salt
pepper
4 tablespoons heavy cream
¼ teaspoon white vinegar
12 chives, chopped

1. Peel the potatoes and cook in salted water until soft. Drain well.
2. Pour the butter into a mixing bowl. Stir in the cornflour (cornstarch), then add the potatoes and mash thoroughly, adding salt and pepper to taste. Leave until cold.
3. Form into a ball and roll out on cornflour (cornstarch) and fit into a 28cm/10 inch flan dish.
4. Blend the cream and vinegar and season with salt and pepper.
5. Pour evenly into the potato case and sprinkle with chives.
6. Bake at 225°C/425°F/Gas mark 7 for 20 to 25 minutes until beginning to brown.

Serve hot with ratatouille, creamed spinach or broccoli spears.

C
W
D — if non-dairy cream and vegetable margarine substituted
Veg

Shallot Pearls

Serves 4

UK

1kg/2 lb shallots or baby onions, peeled
50g/2 oz butter
2 teaspoons sugar
1 teaspoon mustard powder
½ teaspoon salt
¼ teaspoon paprika

US

2 pounds shallots or baby onions, peeled
¼ cup butter
2 teaspoons sugar
1 teaspoon mustard powder
½ teaspoon salt
¼ teaspoon paprika

1. Put the shallots in a large saucepan, just cover with water and simmer for 10 to 15 minutes until tender, basting occasionally. Drain and place in an oven-proof dish.
2. Heat the oven to 180°C/350°F/Gas mark 4.
3. Melt the butter and stir in the remaining ingredients.
4. Pour evenly over the shallots and bake for 30 to 35 minutes, basting occasionally until beginning to brown on top.

C		
W		
D	— if vegetable margarine	substituted
Veg		

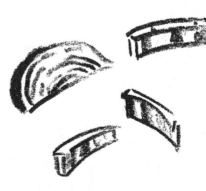

Stuffed Acorn Squash

Serves 4

UK

4 small acorn squash, each about
    285g/10 oz
salt
½ teaspoon Worcestershire or Holbrooks
    sauce
½ teaspoon mustard powder
6 tablespoons curd cheese
25g/1 oz cashew nuts, grated

US

4 small acorn squash, each about 10
    ounces
salt
½ teaspoon Worcestershire or Holbrooks
    sauce
½ teaspoon mustard powder
6 tablespoons farmer's cheese
¼ cup cashew nuts, grated

1. Cook the squash in a large pan of boiling salted water for 15 to 20 minutes until a fork can be easily inserted into the centre.
2. Carefully remove a thick slice from the top of each squash and scoop out and discard the seeds. Remove a thin slice from the bottoms so that the squash will stand upright during baking.
3. Scoop out the flesh and mash with the Worcestershire sauce, mustard and cheese and add salt to taste.
4. Pack into the hollows of the squash and sprinkle with the nuts.
5. Place in a baking dish and bake at 190°C/375°F/Gas mark 5 for 20 to 25 minutes until browned on top.

> Negligible tyramine cheese
> **C**
> **W**
> **D** — if non-dairy cream is
>   substituted

Wrap-roasted Corn

Serves 4

UK

1 cabbage lettuce
4 corn cobs
75g/3 oz butter
1 teaspoon chopped lemon thyme leaves
½ teaspoon marjoram
salt
pepper

US

1 cabbage lettuce
4 corn cobs
⅓ cup butter
1 teaspoon chopped lemon thyme leaves
½ teaspoon marjoram
salt
pepper

1. Wash lettuce and separate leaves.
2. Remove husks and silk from corn.
3. Soften butter and mix in herbs. Spread over corn.
4. Wrap each corn cob in a few lettuce leaves.
5. Place seam sides down in a shallow baking dish in a single layer. Cover tightly with foil.
6. Bake in a preheated oven 230°C/ 450°F/Gas mark 8 for 20 to 25 minutes.
7. Remove lettuce leaves if too tough and serve cobs hot seasoned with salt and pepper.

C
W
D — if vegetable margarine substituted
Veg

DESSERTS AND CAKES

Apple Crunch

Serves 4 to 6

UK

1kg/2 lb cooking apples
50g/2 oz demerara sugar
¼ teaspoon ground cloves
25g/1 oz pumpkin seeds, toasted
100g/4 oz butter
225g/8 oz porridge oats
1 teaspoon ground allspice

US

2 pounds cooking apples
⅓ cup demerara sugar
¼ teaspoon ground cloves
¼ cup pumpkin seeds, toasted
1½ cups butter
2 cups porridge oats
1 teaspoon ground allspice

1. Peel, core and thickly slice the apples.
2. Place in an oven-proof dish. Sprinkle with the sugar and ground cloves mixed together.
3. Stir in the pumpkin seeds.
4. Melt the butter and mix in the porridge oats and allspice.
5. Spoon over the apples and press down lightly.
6. Bake at 160°C/325°F/Gas mark 3 for 25 to 30 minutes until the apples are soft and the topping is crisp.

C
W
D — if vegetable margarine is
    substituted
Veg

Apricot Meringue Pie

Serves 5 to 6

UK

Base

75g/3 oz fine oatmeal
25g/1 oz potato flour
25g/1 oz ground almonds
50g/2 oz soft margarine
1 tablespoon cold water

Filling

1 × 390g/14 oz tin apricots in natural
   juice
3 size 2 egg yolks
40g/1½ oz soft margarine
2 tablespoons caster sugar
2 tablespoons cornflour

Topping

3 size 2 egg whites
pinch cream of tartar
100g/4 oz caster sugar
½ teaspoon vanilla flavouring

US

Base

¾ cup fine oatmeal
3 tablespoons potato flour
¼ cup ground almonds
¼ cup soft margarine
1 tablespoon cold water

Filling

14 ounces canned apricots in natural
   juice
3 large egg yolks
2 tablespoons soft margarine
2 tablespoons superfine sugar
2 tablespoons cornstarch

Topping

3 large egg whites
pinch cream of tartar
½ cup superfine sugar
½ teaspoon vanilla flavoring

Base

1. To make base: mix all ingredients together into a ball. Flatten between sheets of non-stick parchment, then press into base and sides of shallow loose-bottomed 20cm/8 inch fluted flan tin.
2. Bake at 200°C/400°F/Gas mark 6 for about 15 minutes.

Filling

1. Make the filling while pastry is baking: purée all ingredients together in blender [some specks of margarine may not dissolve].
2. Pour into a thick-based saucepan and cook over low heat, stirring continuously until mixture thickens.
3. Pour into pastry case.

Topping

1. To make topping: whisk egg whites and cream of tartar to stiff peaks. Whisk in half the sugar a teaspoonful at a time. Whisk in remaining sugar and vanilla essence to a stiff meringue.
2. Pile meringue on to filling, making sure that the meringue touches the sides of flan tin.
3. Replace pie in oven, reduce heat to 160°C/325°F/Gas mark 3 and bake for 10 to 15 minutes to a pale biscuit colour.

4. Serve warm or cold, removing pie from tin when cool.

C
W
D — if suitable margarine used
Veg

Brazilian Bananas

Serves 4 to 6

UK

50g/2 oz carob bar
15g/½ oz butter
2 tablespoons milk
115g/4 oz soft brown sugar
1 tablespoon golden syrup
½ teaspoon rum flavouring
4 Buckwheat pancakes [see page 127]
4–6 firm bananas
extra butter for frying
whipped cream [optional]

US

2 ounce carob bar
1¼ tablespoons butter
2 tablespoons milk
½ cup soft brown sugar
1 tablespoon golden syrup
½ teaspoon rum flavoring
4 Buckwheat pancakes [see page 127]
4–6 firm bananas
extra butter for frying
whipped cream [optional]

1. Break up the carob and melt with the 15g/½ oz/1¼ tablespoons butter in a basin over a pan of hot water or in the microwave oven.
2. Stir in the milk and when well blended pour into a saucepan.
3. Add the sugar, syrup and rum flavouring.
4. Stir over low heat until the sugar has dissolved, then bring to the boil and cook without stirring for 2–3 minutes or until slightly thickened.
5. Meanwhile warm the pancakes between two plates over a pan of hot water or in the microwave.
6. Peel and sauté the bananas gently in a little butter until tender but not mushy.
7. Roll one banana in each pancake and arrange on a warm serving platter.
8. Coat with rum sauce and a dollop of cream if wished.

W
C
No alcohol
No chocolate
D — if vegetable margarine and plant milk are substituted
Veg

Carob and Walnut Ice-cream

Makes 600ml/1 pint/2½ cups

UK

15g/½ oz carob powder
25g/1 oz caster sugar
2 to 3 tablespoons boiling water
300ml/½ pint milk
1 egg, beaten
½ teaspoon vanilla flavouring
3 tablespoons single cream
50g/2 oz walnuts, chopped
25g/1 oz dried apricots, chopped

US

2 tablespoons carob powder
2 tablespoons superfine sugar
2 to 3 tablespoons boiling water
1¼ cups milk
1 egg, beaten
½ teaspoon vanilla flavouring
3 tablespoons light cream
½ cup English walnuts, chopped
1 tablespoon dried apricots, chopped

1. Blend carob powder and sugar with boiling water.
2. Make up to 300ml/½ pint/1¼ cups with milk. Heat in saucepan until just below boiling point.
3. Beat egg with vanilla flavouring and 1 tablespoon of the remaining cold milk. Pour steaming mixture on to egg, whisking continuously.
4. Return to saucepan and cook over low heat, stirring continuously for 1 minute until sauce just coats the back of a spoon [the consistency is thin].
5. Leave to cool, then stir in cream [the mixture thickens during cooling].
6. Half freeze, then beat in walnuts and apricots. Complete in ice-cream maker or refreeze until firm but not solid.

No chocolate
C
W
D — if non-dairy cream and milk are substituted
Veg

Carob Roulade

Serves 8

UK

175g/6 oz carob bar
3 tablespoons water
4 eggs, separated
150g/5 oz caster sugar
300ml/½ pint double cream
½ teaspoon vanilla flavouring
icing sugar

US

6 ounce carob bar
3 tablespoons water
4 eggs, separated
⅔ cup superfine sugar
1¼ cups heavy cream
½ teaspoon vanilla flavouring
confectioners' sugar

1. Line a 20 × 30 cm/8 × 12 inch Swiss roll tin (jelly roll tin) with non-stick parchment.
2. Break up the carob and place in a saucepan, add the water and heat slowly until melted. Remove from heat.
3. Beat the egg yolks and sugar until creamy and stir into the melted carob.
4. Using grease-free beaters whisk the egg whites until stiff. Stir 1 spoonful into the mixture, then fold in the remainder with a large metal spoon.
5. Turn into the prepared tin and bake at 180°C/350°F/Gas mark 4 for 20 to 25 minutes until just firm.
6. Cover the cake with a well-dampened clean teacloth and refrigerate for 12 hours.
7. Whip the cream with the vanilla flavouring.
8. Carefully remove the cloth and turn out the cake on to non-stick parchment which has been liberally dusted with icing sugar.
9. Peel away the paper covering.
10. Spread the cream over the cake to within 1cm/½ inch of the edges. Roll up from one narrow edge without undue pressure.
11. Lift the roulade on to a serving platter and sift with icing sugar.

Serve thickly sliced with soft summer fruit if wished.

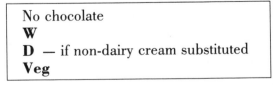

No chocolate
W
D — if non-dairy cream substituted
Veg

Carrot and Pineapple Passion Cake

Serves 6 to 8

UK

2 pineapple rings
225g/8 oz carrots
75g/3 oz butter
150g/5 oz caster sugar
4 eggs, separated
75g/3 oz potato flour
25g/1 oz cornflour
½ teaspoon baking powder
pinch salt
¼ teaspoon ground nutmeg
75g/3 oz very finely chopped pecan nuts
150ml/¼ pint whipped cream

US

2 pineapple rings
1⅓ cup carrots, prepared and finely
   grated
⅓ cup butter
⅔ cup superfine sugar
4 eggs separated
⅔ cup potato flour
¼ cup cornstarch
½ teaspoon baking powder
pinch salt
¼ teaspoon ground nutmeg
⅔ cup very finely chopped pecan nuts
⅔ cup whipped cream

1. Reserve one pineapple ring for
   decoration and finely chop the other.

2. Finely grate the carrots, turn on to
   paper towel and press to remove
   excess moisture.
3. Beat the butter and sugar together in
   a mixing bowl, then gradually beat in
   the egg yolks.
4. Sift in the potato flour, cornflour
   (cornstarch), baking powder, salt and
   nutmeg.
5. Stir in the chopped pineapple, carrot
   and nuts.
6. Using grease-free beaters, whisk the
   egg whites to stiff peaks. Fold into
   the mixture.
7. Pour into a well-greased 20cm/7 inch
   round cake tin and bake at 180°C/
   350°F/Gas mark 4 for 45 minutes to
   1 hour until a skewer inserted into
   the centre comes out clean. Lower
   the temperature during cooking if the
   cake is becoming too brown.
8. Cool the cake on a wire rack, then
   decorate with rosettes of cream and
   the reserved pineapple ring cut into
   small wedges.

C
No chocolate
W
D — if soya flour and non-dairy
      cream substituted
Veg

Fruited Tapioca Pudding

Serves 4 to 5

UK

50g/2 oz tapioca
450ml/¾ pint milk
¼ teaspoon ground nutmeg
1 × 225g/8 oz tin pineapple rings in
    natural juice
1 × 275g/10 oz tin gooseberries
25g/1 oz sugar

US

½ cup tapioca
2 cups milk
¼ teaspoon ground nutmeg
8 ounces canned pineapple rings in
    natural juice
10 ounces canned gooseberries
2 tablespoons sugar

1. Put tapioca and milk and nutmeg in saucepan.
2. Drain fruit, reserving juice. Add 150ml/¼ pint/⅔ cup of the juice to the pan.
3. Cook over low heat for 15 minutes or until mixture thickens, stirring frequently.
4. Mix in sugar and fruit.
5. Transfer to a greased 1.2 litre/2 pint/5 cup pie dish.
6. Bake at 200°C/400°F/Gas mark 6 for 25 to 35 minutes until a pale biscuit colour.
7. Serve hot.

W
C
D — if soya milk substituted
Veg

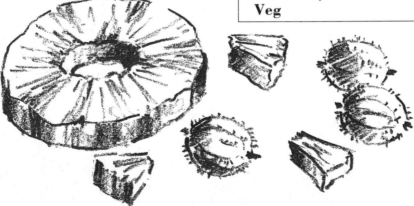

Kiwi Soufflé

Serves 6

UK

3 kiwi fruit
3 tablespoons apple juice
3 tablespoons water
2 tablespoons powdered gelatine
100g/4 oz sugar
4 eggs, separated
300ml/½ pint whipping cream, half-
   whipped
25g/1 oz carob bar, grated and chilled

US

3 kiwi fruit
3 tablespoons apple juice
3 tablespoons water
2 tablespoons powdered gelatine
½ cup sugar
4 eggs, separated
1¼ cups whipping cream, half whipped
25g/1 oz carob bar, grated and chilled

1. Fold a long sheet of foil in half along length and wrap around a 15-cm/6-inch soufflé dish to form a collar that protrudes above the rim. Overlap ends and secure at top.
2. Peel and mash the kiwi fruit and press through a nylon sieve to remove seeds if wished.
3. Mix the apple juice, water, gelatine or agar-agar and sugar in a saucepan and heat gently, stirring until dissolved. Raise the heat and bring to the boil.
4. Leave to stand for 2 minutes. Beat the egg yolks with 2 extra teaspoons cold water and strain in to the hot syrup.
5. Return pan to very low heat and cook stirring continuously for 1 minute. Overcooking will cause curdling.
6. Pour into a mixing bowl, cover and cool. Mix in the sieved kiwi fruit.
7. When almost set, fold in the cream.
8. Using grease-free beaters, whisk the egg whites to stiff peaks. Fold into the mixture.
9. Pour into the prepared soufflé dish and chill for 4 hours.
10. Remove foil collar with the aid of a warmed table knife and decorate the top with grated carob bar.

C
W
D — if non-dairy cream substituted
Veg — if agar-agar used instead of
         gelatine

Pecan Pie

Serves 5 to 6

UK

Base

75g/3 oz fine oatmeal
25g/1 oz potato flour
25g/1 oz ground almonds
50g/2 oz soft margarine
1 tablespoon cold water

Filling

2 eggs
150g/5 oz soft brown sugar
pinch salt
75g/3 oz soft margarine
120ml/4 fl oz corn syrup
75g/3 oz pecan nuts

US

Base

¾ cup fine oatmeal
3 tablespoons potato flour
¼ cup ground almonds
¼ cup soft margarine
1 tablespoon cold water

Filling

2 eggs
1 cup soft brown sugar
pinch salt
⅓ cup soft margarine
⅓ cup corn syrup
⅔ cup pecan nuts

1. Mix base ingredients together to form a ball. Press out into base and sides of a well-greased 18-cm/7-inch flan tin. Chill for 10 minutes.
2. Pre-heat oven to 190°C/375°F/Gas mark 5.
3. Bake pastry for 10 minutes.
4. Meanwhile beat the eggs, sugar, salt, margarine and syrup together thoroughly with a wooden spoon.
5. Coarsely break about half the pecans and stir into the mixture with the remaining pecans.
6. Pour into the flan case. Reduce the heat to 180°C/350°F/Gas mark 4 and bake for 35 to 40 minutes, covering the pie with foil if the pastry begins to brown too much.

Serve warm or cold with whipped cream.

For added nutrition substitute toasted sunflower seeds for 25g/1oz/¼ cup of the pecans.

No chocolate
C
W
D — if vegetable margarine and non-dairy cream are substituted
Veg

Redcurrant and Peach Pavlova

Serves 6 to 7

UK

3 egg whites
200g/7 oz caster sugar
2 teaspoons cornflour ⎫
½ teaspoon vanilla flavouring ⎬ blended together
1 teaspoon white malt vinegar ⎭

Topping

1 × 390/14 oz tin peach slices in syrup
50g/2 oz redcurrants, rinsed and
  trimmed
150ml/¼ pint whipping cream, whipped

US

3 egg whites
1 cup superfine sugar
2 teaspoons cornstarch ⎫
½ teaspoon vanilla flavoring ⎬ blended together
1 teaspoon white malt vinegar ⎭

Topping

14 ounces canned peach slices in syrup
⅓ cup redcurrants, rinsed and trimmed
⅔ cup whipping cream, whipped

1. Pre-heat oven to 150°C/300°F/Gas mark 2.
2. Whisk egg whites to stiff peaks in a grease-free bowl.
3. Whisk in sugar gradually until stiff, then beat in blended cornflour (cornstarch).
4. Continue beating until mixture is heavy and smooth.
5. Place sheet of baking parchment on baking tray.
6. Spoon mixture into centre and spread gently to a round 2.5cm/1 inch thick.
7. Place on middle shelf and bake 30 minutes, then reduce heat to 140°C/275°F/Gas mark 1 for a further 30 minutes. Switch off oven but do not open door until meringue is cool [about 1 hour].
8. Meanwhile drain peach slices into a saucepan. Reserve peaches.
9. Add redcurrants to pan and poach until softened. Remove with slotted spoon, then simmer syrup until only 2 tablespoons liquid remains.
10. To serve, arrange peach slices in cartwheel fashion on meringue, decorate with redcurrants, then pour on syrup to glaze.
11. Serve with cream.

```
C
W
D — if cream omitted or non-dairy
    cream substituted
Veg
```

Vanilla and Carob Swirl Cheesecake

Serves 6

UK

120g/4½ oz caster sugar
225g/8 oz fromage frais
1 tablespoon cornflour
1 egg, beaten
2 drops almond essence
½ teaspoon vanilla flavouring
30g/1 oz carob powder
20-cm/8-inch almond and oatmeal part-
  baked pastry case [see page 122]

US

½ cup caster sugar
1 cup fromage frais
1 tablespoon cornstarch
1 egg, beaten
2 drops almond essence
½ teaspoon vanilla flavoring
¼ cup carob powder
8-inch almond and oatmeal part baked
  pastry case [see page 122]

1. Beat three quarters of the sugar with the fromage frais and cornflour (cornstarch) until heavy and smooth.
2. Add the egg, almond essence and vanilla flavouring and continue beating to a thick batter.
3. Set aside about one quarter of the mixture.
4. Mix the carob with the remaining sugar and stir into the larger quantity of filling.
5. Place the pastry case on a baking tray and pour in the carob filling. Top with the reserved vanilla filling then swirl through with a fork to achieve a marbling effect.
6. Bake in the centre of the oven at 180°C/350°F/Gas mark 4 for 30 to 45 minutes until the centre is no longer wobbly.
7. Leave to cool, then refrigerate for at least 4 hours.

> **W**
> No chocolate
> **C**
> Negligible tyramine cheese
> **Veg**

BISCUITS AND SWEETMEATS

Almond bars

Makes 15 bars

UK

100g/4 oz butter
100g/4 oz caster sugar
2 eggs, beaten
3 drops almond flavouring
100g/4 oz potato flour
50g/2 oz ground almonds
50g/2 oz flaked almonds

US

1 cup butter
½ cup superfine sugar
2 eggs, beaten
3 drops almond flavoring
¾ cup potato flour
½ cup ground almonds
½ cup slivered almonds

1. Beat butter and sugar together until fluffy.
2. Add beaten eggs and almond flavouring a little at a time, beating thoroughly in between each addition.
3. Mix in potato flour and ground almonds.
4. Spoon into a 19-cm/7½-inch square shallow tin. Smooth the top and sprinkle with flaked (slivered) almonds.
5. Bake in a pre-heated oven 200°C/400°F/Gas mark 6 for 15 minutes until set and golden in colour.
6. Leave to cool before cutting into bars with a sharp knife.

W
C
D — if vegetable margarine is substituted
Veg

Brownies

Makes 16

UK

100g/4 oz butter or margarine
25g/1 oz carob powder
½ teaspoon vanilla flavouring
2 eggs
175g/6 oz soft brown sugar
50g/2 oz self-raising flour
¼ teaspoon baking powder
pinch salt
50g/2 oz chopped mixed nuts
150g/5 oz carob bars or carob drops

US

1 cup butter or margarine
¼ cup carob powder
½ teaspoon vanilla flavoring
2 eggs
⅔ cup soft brown sugar
½ cup self-rising flour
¼ teaspoon baking powder
pinch salt
½ cup chopped mixed nuts
5 ounce carob bar or carob drops

1. Lightly grease and flour a 20-cm/8-inch square shallow cake tin.
2. Melt the butter and stir in the carob powder and vanilla flavouring.
3. Beat the eggs until foamy, then beat in the sugar.
4. Sieve the flour, baking powder and salt on to the mixture and stir in gently.
5. Pour in the melted butter and carob and mix thoroughly but lightly. Stir in the nuts.
6. Spoon mixture into prepared cake tin and bake at 180°C/350°F/Gas mark 5 for 25 to 35 minutes until a skewer inserted into the centre comes out clean.
7. Leave in tin until cool.
8. Melt carob bars or drops in a bowl over a pan of hot water.
9. Pour over brownies and cut into squares when set.

No chocolate
C
D — if vegetable margarine is substituted
Veg

Carob Coconut Pyramids

Makes 12 to 16

UK

225g/8 oz desiccated coconut
100g/4 oz caster sugar
40g/1½ oz rice flour
1 tablespoon carob powder
½ teaspoon vanilla flavouring
3 egg whites
2 to 4 sheets rice paper
6 to 8 glacé cherries, halved

US

2½ cups desiccated coconut
½ cup superfine sugar
⅓ cup rice flour
1 tablespoon carob powder
½ teaspoon vanilla flavoring
3 egg whites
2 to 4 sheets rice paper
6 to 8 glacé cherries, halved

1. Combine coconut, sugar, rice flour and carob.
2. Whisk vanilla flavouring with egg white to soft peaks.
3. Fold egg whites into dry mixture.
4. With dampened hands, form mixture into 12 pyramids.
5. Place on baking sheets lined with rice paper.
6. Bake at 150°C/300°F/Gas mark 2 for 30 to 40 minutes until just firm.
7. Loosen rice paper from baking trays with palette knife.
8. Top pyramids with cherries.

> No chocolate
> **W**
> **C**
> **D**
> **Veg**

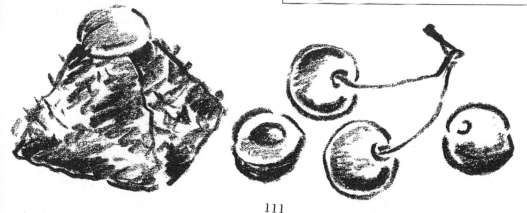

Date and Almond Crunchies

Makes 24

UK

rice paper
2 egg whites
200g/7 oz caster sugar
1 teaspoon golden syrup
225g/8 oz ground almonds
50g/2 oz stoned or block dates, chopped

US

rice paper
2 egg whites
1 cup superfine sugar
1 teaspoon golden syrup
2 cups ground almonds
½ cup pitted or block dates, chopped

1. Line two baking trays with rice paper.
2. In a grease-free bowl, whisk egg whites to stiff peaks.
3. Whisk in sugar a little at a time, then add syrup and whisk until stiff.
4. Fold in ground almonds and dates.
5. Place small mounds of mixture well spaced out on to lined baking trays.
6. Bake at 160°C/325°F/Gas mark 3 for 20 minutes or until golden brown.
7. Slide a palette knife between rice paper and baking tray to loosen, then remove, cool on wire rack and trim off rice paper.

W
D
C
Veg

Florentines

Makes 8

UK

40g/1½ oz vegetable margarine
50g/2 oz soft brown sugar
50g/2 oz flaked almonds
25g/1 oz seedless raisins, coarsely
   chopped
100g/3½ oz carob bar

US

3¾ tablespoons vegetable margarine
¼ cup soft brown sugar
½ cup slivered almonds
3 tablespoons seedless raisins, coarsely
   chopped
3½ ounce carob bar

```
W
D
No chocolate
C
Vegan
```

1. Melt the margarine in a heavy-based saucepan over low heat.
2. Stir in the sugar until dissolved. Raise the heat until the mixture bubbles.
3. Stir in the almonds and raisins and immediately remove from the heat.
4. Line two baking trays with non-stick parchment.
5. Place 4 teaspoons of the mixture on each, making sure that they are well spaced out as the biscuits spread during baking.
6. Bake at 180°C/350°F/Gas mark 4 for 10 to 12 minutes until light brown.
7. Leave until crisp, then remove with a palette knife and reverse on to a wire rack.
8. Meanwhile break up the carob bar and melt in a basin over a pan of hot water or in the microwave.
9. Spoon the melted carob over the biscuits and mark in a zig-zag pattern with a fork before completely set.

Marzipan Dates

Makes 16

UK

16 fresh dates
50g/2 oz white marzipan
1 tablespoon finely chopped pistachio
    nuts

US

16 fresh dates
½ cup white marzipan
1 tablespoon finely chopped pistachio
    nuts

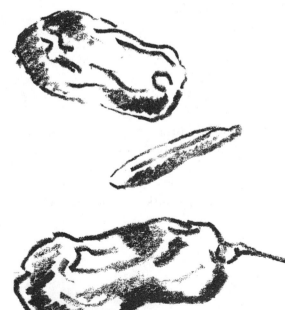

1. Make a long slit lengthways in the dates and remove the stones (pits).
2. Divide the marzipan into 16 pieces and roll into tiny sausage shapes [lightly dust the palms of the hands with icing sugar or cornflour (cornstarch) before shaping].
3. Stuff the dates with the marzipan and press a few chopped pistachio nuts along the exposed side of the marzipan.
4. Arrange on a dish lined with a paper doily.

When buying commercial marzipan make sure that the ingredients are suitable.

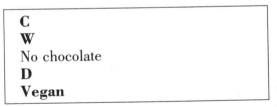

C
W
No chocolate
D
Vegan

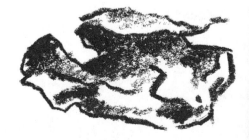

New Moon Peanut Crisps

Makes 15 to 20

UK

75g/3 oz shelled peanuts, skinned
75g/3 oz demerara sugar
few drops vanilla flavouring
2–3 teaspoons beaten egg
50g/2 oz carob drops
4 drops sunflower oil

US

⅔ cup shelled peanuts, skinned
½ cup demerara sugar
few drops vanilla flavoring
2–3 teaspoons beaten egg
6 tablespoons carob drops
4 drops safflower oil

1. Finely grind the peanuts in the blender.
2. Add the sugar, vanilla flavouring and sufficient egg to mix to a firm paste. Gather into a ball with hands dusted with cornflour (cornstarch) and divide mixture in half.
3. Roll out one piece between 2 sheets of non-stick parchment to a 2-mm/⅛-inch thickness. Lightly oil the edge of a 3-cm/1½-inch pastry cutter and cut out as many rounds as possible. Remove the trimmings.
4. Space out biscuits. They will not spread very much during cooking. Carefully lift both lining and biscuits on to a large baking sheet.
5. Roll the remaining mixture and trimmings in the same way and transfer to a baking sheet.
6. Bake at 180°C/350°F/Gas mark 4 for 10 to 12 minutes until light brown. Remove from oven and leave to cool.
7. Melt the carob drops in a basin over a pan of hot water or in the microwave oven. Stir in the oil.
8. Dip one edge of each biscuit in the melted carob and place on the cooled baking trays and leave until set.

W
D
No chocolate
Vegan

Rice Paper Sandwiches

Makes 16

UK

50g/2 oz raisins
50g/2 oz currants
50g/2 oz dried apricots
25g/1 oz sultanas
100g/4 oz stoned dates
25g/1 oz walnut halves
1 teaspoon clear honey
Few sheets of rice paper

US

⅓ cup raisins
⅓ cup currants
⅓ cup dried apricots
¼ cup golden seedless raisins
½ cup pitted dates
⅓ cup English walnut halves
1 teaspoon clear honey
Few sheets of rice paper

1. Cover the back of a baking tray with rice paper, overlapping sheets if necessary.
2. Mince the fruits and walnuts.
3. Add the honey and work to a stiff smooth paste.
4. Using a warmed damp table knife, carefully spread the mixture over rice paper. Cover with rice paper and apply light pressure with a rolling pin to flatten filling evenly.
5. Cut into 16 bars with a sharp knife.
6. Without covering, refrigerate for at least 1 hour to help the filling to harden.

Serve as a snack or sweetmeat.

These sweetmeats will keep for 1 to 2 weeks in a covered container in the refrigerator or cool place.

| C |
| W |
| D |
| No chocolate |

Rum Truffles

Makes 16 to 20

UK

2 × 100g/3½ oz carob bars
25g/1 oz butter
few drops rum essence
2 drops vanilla flavouring
1 tablespoon single cream
2 egg yolks
1–2 tablespoons carob powder

US

2 × 3½ ounce carob bars
2½ tablespoons butter
few drops rum essence
2 drops vanilla flavoring
1 tablespoon light cream
2 egg yolks
1–2 tablespoons carob powder

1. Break up the carob bars and put into a large bowl over a pan of hot water or melt in the microwave.
2. When melted, add the butter, rum and vanilla flavouring, cream and beaten egg yolks.
3. Stir continuously until thickened.
4. Remove from heat and divide mixture and shape into small balls.
5. Leave until firm, then toss in the carob powder.

No chocolate
W
No alcohol
D — if vegetable margarine and
    milk are substituted
Veg

Spiced Carob Cookies

Makes 12 to 15

UK

100g/4 oz ground almonds
100g/4 oz caster sugar
1 teaspoon cinnamon
½ teaspoon ground nutmeg
1 tablespoon carob powder
2 egg whites
icing sugar

US

1 cup ground almonds
½ cup superfine sugar
1 teaspoon cinnamon
½ teaspoon ground nutmeg
1 tablespoon carob powder
2 egg whites
confectioners' sugar

1. Sift the ground almonds, sugar, cinnamon, nutmeg and carob into a mixing bowl.
2. Whisk the egg whites to soft peaks and fold into the mixture.
3. Divide into walnut-sized pieces and shape into soft balls with dampened hands.
4. Place spaced out on a well-greased or non-stick parchment-lined baking tray.
5. Bake at 180°C/350°F/Gas mark 4 for 25 to 30 minutes until the cookies can be removed easily from the tray with a palette knife.
6. Cool on a wire rack and dust with icing sugar.

```
W
D
No chocolate
C
Veg
```

Walnut Fudge

Makes 750g/1½ lb but keeps in an
airtight container if the layers are
interleaved with greaseproof paper

UK

150ml/¼ pint evaporated milk
150ml/¼ pint milk
50g/2 oz butter
450g/1 lb caster sugar
1 teaspoon vanilla flavouring
25g/1 oz chopped walnuts

US

⅔ cup evaporated milk
⅔ cup milk
¼ cup butter
2 cups superfine sugar
1 teaspoon vanilla flavoring
3 tablespoons chopped English walnuts

1. Grease a 19-cm/7½-inch shallow
    square cake tin.
2. Have ready a glass of cold water.
3. Combine the evaporated and fresh
    milk, butter, sugar and vanilla
    flavouring in a heavy-based
    saucepan.
4. Cook over low heat, stirring
    occasionally, until the butter melts
    and the sugar dissolves.
5. Without further stirring, raise the
    heat, bring to the boil and cook

rapidly to 115°C/238°F when a few
drops of the syrup form a soft ball
when dropped into cold water.
6. Immediately draw the pan away from
    the heat to prevent further cooking.
7. Add the walnuts and beat the
    mixture with a wooden spoon until it
    thickens.
8. Pour into the prepared tin, leave for
    a few minutes to cool down, then
    mark into squares.
9. Remove from tin when completely
    cold and cut the fudge into squares.

No chocolate
C
W
D — if vegetable margarine and
concentrated plant milk are
substituted for butter and milk
Veg

SAUCES, PASTRY AND OTHERS

Béchamel Sauce

Makes 300ml/½ pint/1¼ cups

UK

300ml/½ pint milk
1 slice onion
1 slice carrot
1 bay leaf
1 blade mace
3 sprigs parsley
1 sprig thyme
6 peppercorns
20g/¾ oz butter
20g/¾ oz cornflour
salt
pepper

US

1¼ cups milk
1 slice onion
1 slice carrot
1 bay leaf
1 blade mace
3 sprigs parsley
1 sprig thyme
6 peppercorns

1½ tablespoons butter
3 tablespoons cornstarch
salt
pepper

1. Put the milk, onion, carrot, bay leaf, mace, parsley, thyme and peppercorns in a saucepan.
2. Heat until steaming but not boiling. Cover with the lid and switch off heat. Leave to infuse for 30 minutes.
3. Melt the butter in a saucepan. Draw pan away from heat and stir in cornflour (cornstarch).
4. Strain in milk and stir until smooth.
5. Place pan over medium heat and bring to the boil, stirring continuously. Reduce heat and cook, still stirring, for 3 to 4 minutes. Season with salt and pepper.

> **W**
> **D** — if vegetable margarine and milk substituted
> **Veg**

Mushroom Sauce

Makes about 200ml/7 fl oz/⅞ cup

UK

225g/8 oz mushrooms, finely chopped
3 spring onions, trimmed and finely
   sliced
15ml/1 tablespoon olive oil
1 teaspoon arrowroot
2 tablespoons grape juice
salt
freshly ground black pepper
1 tablespoon freshly chopped parsley

US

3 cups mushrooms, finely chopped
3 scallions, trimmed and finely sliced
1 tablespoon olive oil
1 teaspoon arrowroot
2 tablespoons grape juice
salt
freshly ground black pepper
1 tablespoon freshly chopped parsley

1. Gently fry the mushrooms and onions in the oil until the mushroom juices have almost evaporated.
2. Blend arrowroot and grape juice.
3. Stir into mushrooms and onions and cook over low heat, stirring. continuously until thickened. Season with salt and pepper to taste.
4. Stir in parsley.
5. Serve hot, adding extra water if reheating.

W
C
D
No wine
Veg

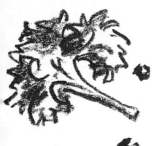
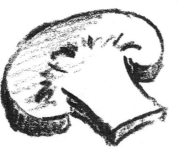
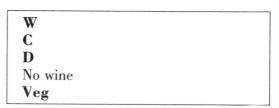

Almond and Oatmeal Pastry

Enough to fit an 18-cm/7-inch flan tin or dish [a loose-bottomed tin is recommended.]

A pastry that is relatively easy to handle, it can be rolled out to fit a 15–18cm/6–7 inch flan dish without having to do too much patching. It can also be used as a pie crust. The baked pastry is a warm golden colour, the flavour is neutral and the texture crisp. It is suitable for both sweet and savoury fillings and can double as a crumb crust which is a consideration as most commercially produced biscuits are made with wheat. Bake at 200°C/400°F/Gas mark 6 for 10 minutes if the filling is not to be further cooked, otherwise bake for 5 minutes, add filling and continue cooking at the temperature and required time called for by the recipe.

UK

100g/4 oz ground almonds
75g/3 oz fine oatmeal
50g/2 oz butter

US

1 cup ground almonds
¾ cup fine oatmeal
¼ cup butter

1. Mix the almonds and oatmeal together, add the butter and mix to a smooth paste. Gather into a ball and roll out on cornflour (cornstarch). Use as required.

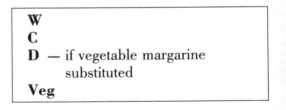

W
C
D — if vegetable margarine
       substituted
Veg

Brazil Nut and Brown Rice Pastry

Enough for 1 ×18-cm/7-inch flan case or 3 × 7-cm/3½-inch individual tartlet cases.

A very sturdy pastry which holds its shape well making it ideal for use in flans and tarts that are un-moulded. First bake the pastry case at 190°C/375°F/Gas mark 5 for 10 minutes. Leave to cool down, then remove from tin, fill as required and continue baking according to the recipe. If pastry case is to be filled and served without additional baking, allow 15 to 20 minutes total cooking time. The appearance is similar to wholewheat pastry and although it can be used with sweet fillings, it goes particularly well with savoury fillings. Roll out on cornflour (cornstarch) and press into flan cases or lift carefully if using as a top crust.

UK

40g/1½ oz Brazil nut flour [or nuts of your choice finely ground]
125g/4 oz brown rice flour
¼ level teaspoon agar-agar
2 tablespoons sunflower oil
4 tablespoons cold water

US

⅓ cup Brazil nut flour [or nuts of your choice finely ground]
¾ cup brown rice flour
¼ teaspoon agar-agar
2 tablespoons safflower oil
4 tablespoons cold water

1. Thoroughly mix the dry ingredients, then add the oil and water and mix to a manageable dough. Use as required.

W
C
D
Vegan

Brown Rice and Cornflour Pastry

Enough for 1 × 18-cm/8-inch flan case

An excellent flavour, this pastry also has a good crisp texture and traditional pastry colour when baked. Use for flan cases which are to be served directly from the flan dish or tin. Bake at 190°C/375°F/Gas mark 5 for 10 minutes if baking is to be continued after filling. If using with a cooked filling allow 15 to 20 minutes for complete cooking. The pastry is best pressed into the tin rather than rolled out but can be used as a pie crust in the following way:

First roll out on cornflour (cornstarch), then using a 2.5–5-cm/1–2-inch pastry cutter cut out as many coin-shaped pieces as possible, re-rolling the pastry trimmings. Brush the edges of the pastry circles with water, milk or beaten egg and place overlapped on top of the filling, making sure there are no gaps.

UK

175g/6 oz cornflour
175g/6 oz brown rice flour
85g/3 oz soya margarine
2 teaspoons cold water

US

1½ cups cornstarch
1 cup brown rice flour
⅓ cup soya margarine
2 teaspoons cold water

1. Mix the cornflour (cornstarch) and brown rice flour together and rub in the margarine. Add the water and mix to a soft dough. Use as required.

W
C
D
Vegan

Cornflour and Potato Flour Pastry

Enough for 1 × 18-cm/7-inch flan case or 3 × 7-cm/3½-inch individual tartlet cases

Do not be put off by the title, this is quite the most delicious short pastry that melts in the mouth and is as light as air. Although delicate, this pastry can be turned out easily and it is equally good with either savoury or sweet fillings. When baked the pastry retains its pale colour. Press into the dish or tin to prepare flan cases, but although the pastry rolls out well, it may crack as it is transferred to cover a pie. You may find it easier to use small pastry cutters to make an overlapping design [see Brown Rice and Cornflour Pastry, page 124] or having rolled the pastry out on cornflour (cornstarch), cut into 4 wedges, then place individually on top of the filling and pinch the joins together rather like the finish on a Cornish pasty [see diag].

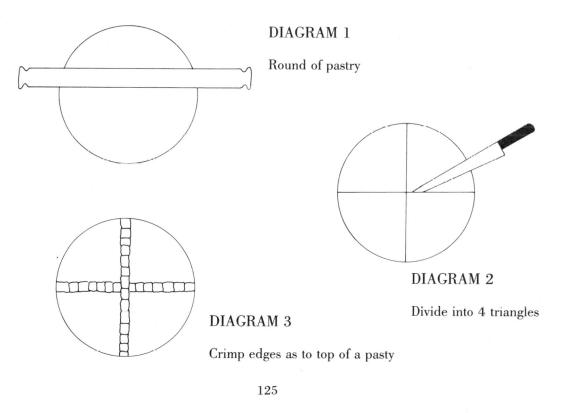

DIAGRAM 1

Round of pastry

DIAGRAM 2

Divide into 4 triangles

DIAGRAM 3

Crimp edges as to top of a pasty

Bake at 200C/400F/Gas mark 6 for 5 minutes if proceeding to bake after filling. Allow 10 to 15 minutes to bake completely if filling just before serving.

UK

100g/4 oz cornflour
50g/2 oz potato flour [Farina]
pinch salt
75g/3 oz soya margarine
4 teaspoons cold water

US

1 cup cornstarch
½ cup potato flour [Farina]
pinch salt
⅓ cup soya margarine
4 teaspoons cold water

1. Combine all the ingredients in the blender and mix to a smooth paste or mix the dry ingredients together in a bowl, rub in the margarine and stir in the water. Shape into a soft ball and roll out on cornflour (cornstarch).

W
C
D
Vegan

Buckwheat Pancakes

Makes 6 to 10

UK

50g/2 oz buckwheat flour
50g/2 oz cornflour
25g/1 oz fine oatmeal
½ teaspoon salt
1 teaspoon bicarbonate of soda
2 teaspoons cream of tartar
4 tablespoons sunflower oil
1 large egg
300ml/½ pint milk
1 tablespoon molasses
extra oil for frying

US

½ cup buckwheat flour
½ cup cornstarch
¼ cup fine oatmeal
½ teaspoon salt
1 teaspoon baking soda
2 teaspoons cream of tartar
4 tablespoons safflower oil
1 large egg
1¼ cups milk
1 tablespoon molasses
extra oil for frying

W	
C	
D	— if soya milk substituted
Veg	

1. Sieve the dry ingredients into a mixing bowl.
2. Beat in the remaining ingredients with a wire whisk until the mixture is smooth.
3. Leave to stand for 15 to 20 minutes, then stir with the whisk to achieve a smooth batter which should be the consistency of cream.
4. Lightly oil a non-stick omelette or frying pan (skillet), place over heat and, when hot, pour in two or three tablespoons batter [depending on size of pan used]. Tip pan to spread batter evenly and when nearly set, draw pan away from heat, turn pancake over and return to heat to cook the other side.
5. Repeat with remaining batter. Stack and keep pancakes warm or freeze cooled pancakes, interleaved with non-stick parchment and overwrapped in freezer film.

Buckwheat pancakes known as crêpes blé noir originated in Brittany. The texture is very soft but the pancakes are thicker than 'crêpes' and light brown in colour.

Suitable for sweet or savoury fillings.

Cooked Mayonnaise

Makes about 300ml/½ pint/1¼ cups

UK

1 tablespoon flour
2 teaspoons caster sugar
1 teaspoon salt
1 teaspoon mustard powder
3 tablespoons cider vinegar
5 tablespoons cold water
15g/½ oz butter or margarine
1 large egg
5 tablespoons single cream

US

1 tablespoon flour
2 teaspoons superfine sugar
1 teaspoon salt
1 teaspoon mustard powder
3 tablespoons cider vinegar
5 tablespoons cold water
1¼ tablespoons butter or margarine
1 large egg
5 tablespoons light cream

1. In a small saucepan, blend together the flour, sugar, salt, mustard, vinegar and water.
2. When the mixture is smooth, place saucepan over low heat and cook, stirring continuously, for 5 minutes.
3. Stir in butter.
4. Beat the egg with 1 further tablespoon water and 2 tablespoons of the hot sauce.
5. Pour into the sauce and heat gently until very hot but not boiling, beating vigorously with a whisk.
6. Pour into a bowl and cool rapidly.
7. Stir cream into sauce when cold.

In this recipe the egg is cooked, making the mayonnaise suitable for those not wishing to use 'raw-egg' mayonnaise.

> **C**
> **D** — if vegetable margarine and non-dairy cream substituted
> **Veg**

Dill Weed Sauce

Makes 150ml/¼ pint/⅔ cup

UK

1 egg yolk
pinch dry mustard
generous pinch salt
generous shake freshly ground black
  pepper
1 tablespoon dill weed leaves
150ml/¼ pint sunflower oil
1 teaspoon white malt vinegar

US

1 egg yolk
pinch dry mustard
generous pinch salt
generous shake freshly ground black
  pepper
1 tablespoon dill weed leaves
⅔ cup safflower oil
1 teaspoon white malt vinegar

1. In a small bowl, beat egg yolk,
   mustard, salt, pepper and dill weed
   with a whisk until creamy.
2. Slowly beat in oil drop by drop until
   mixture becomes thicker.
3. Beat in remaining oil more quickly,
   adding vinegar as sauce continues to
   thicken.

Use eggs only from salmonella-free
chickens and serve freshly made.

C
W
D
Veg

Sauce Gribiche

Makes 200ml/7 fl oz/⅞ cup

UK

yolks of 4 hard-boiled eggs
1 tablespoon French mustard
¼ teaspoon salt
¼ teaspoon freshly ground black pepper
250ml/8 fl oz sunflower oil
1 teaspoon white vinegar
1 teaspoon freshly chopped tarragon
  leaves
1 teaspoon freshly chopped parsley
1 teaspoon freshly chopped chives

US

yolks of 4 hard-cooked eggs
1 tablespoon French mustard
¼ teaspoon salt
¼ teaspoon freshly ground black pepper
1 cup safflower oil
1 teaspoon white vinegar
1 teaspoon freshly chopped tarragon
  leaves
1 teaspoon freshly chopped parsley
1 teaspoon freshly chopped chives

1. Switch on the blender at high speed and feed in the egg yolks, mustard, salt and pepper and 1 teaspoon of the oil.
2. When well blended and while the motor is still running, gradually pour in the remaining oil and blend to a smooth consistency.
3. Add the vinegar and herbs.
4. Use immediately or return to the blender if sauce has separated on standing.

Use in place of mayonnaise when 'raw eggs' are unsuitable.
Those on a low-cholesterol diet should use this sauce sparingly.

C
D
Veg

French Dressing

Makes 300ml/½ pint/1¼ cups

UK

75ml/5 tablespoons white malt vinegar
225ml/8 fl oz corn oil
½ teaspoon caster sugar
1 teaspoon salt
¼ teaspoon freshly ground black pepper
1 teaspoon French mustard

US

⅓ cup white malt vinegar
1 cup corn oil
½ teaspoon superfine sugar
1 teaspoon salt
¼ teaspoon freshly ground black pepper
1 teaspoon French mustard

1. Combine all ingredients in a screwtop jar or well-corked wine bottle and shake vigorously before each use.

Keeps well.

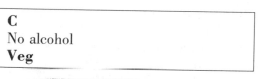

C
No alcohol
Veg

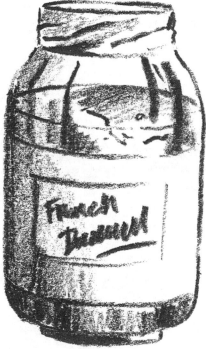

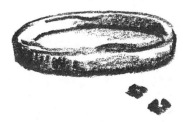

Tomato Chutney

Makes enough for 2 jars

UK

175g/6 oz tomatoes
100g/4 oz shallots
2 green dessert apples
175g/6 oz seedless raisins
100g/4 oz demerara sugar
½ teaspoon cayenne pepper
300ml/½ pint malt vinegar
½ teaspoon salt
3 cloves
1 fresh green chilli

US

175g/6 ounce tomatoes
100g/4 ounce shallots
2 green dessert apples
1 cup seedless raisins
½ cup demerara sugar
½ teaspoon cayenne pepper
1¼ cups malt vinegar
½ teaspoon salt
3 cloves
1 fresh green chilli

1. Peel the tomatoes and shallots. Peel and core the apples.
2. Mince or very finely chop the tomatoes, shallots, apples and raisins.
3. Place in a heavy-based saucepan over very low heat with sugar and cayenne. Cover and cook, stirring frequently, for 15 minutes or until the sugar has dissolved.
4. Add vinegar, salt, cloves and chillies tied in a small piece of clean muslin [or laundered white J cloth].
5. Cook uncovered for 35 to 40 minutes, stirring frequently, until soft and thick.
6. Pour into hot jars sealed and covered with a plastic lid.
7. Serve with cold meat and salad.

C
D
W
Vegan

Tomato Curry Sauce

Makes 300ml/½ pint/1¼ cups

UK

25g/1 oz butter or margarine
1 onion, finely chopped
1 teaspoon curry powder
¼ teaspoon Dijon mustard
¼ teaspoon ground cumin
50g/2 oz mushrooms, chopped
1 × 390g/14 oz tin tomatoes
1 teaspoon malt vinegar
salt
pepper

US

2½ tablespoons butter or margarine
1 onion, finely chopped
1 teaspoon curry powder
¼ teaspoon Dijon mustard
¼ teaspoon ground cumin
¾ cup mushrooms, chopped
1 × 14½ ounce can tomatoes
1 teaspoon malt vinegar
salt
pepper

1. Melt the butter and gently fry the onion until soft.
2. Add curry powder, mustard and cumin and cook, stirring, for 1 minute.
3. Add mushrooms, cook gently for 1 minute, then mix in tomatoes and vinegar and cook over low heat for 15 to 20 minutes.
4. Crush with a potato masher or blend sauce to a purée.
5. Season to taste with salt and pepper.

C
W
No wine
D — if vegetable margarine is
    substituted
Veg

Vinaigrette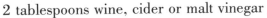

Makes 150ml/¼ pint/⅔ cup

UK & US

2 tablespoons wine, cider or malt vinegar
6 tablespoons olive or sunflower
    (safflower) oil
¼ teaspoon salt
¼ teaspoon freshly ground black pepper
¼ teaspoon, chopped tarragon, chives or
    mixed herbs [optional]

Combine all ingredients and beat
thoroughly before using.

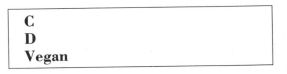

C
D
Vegan

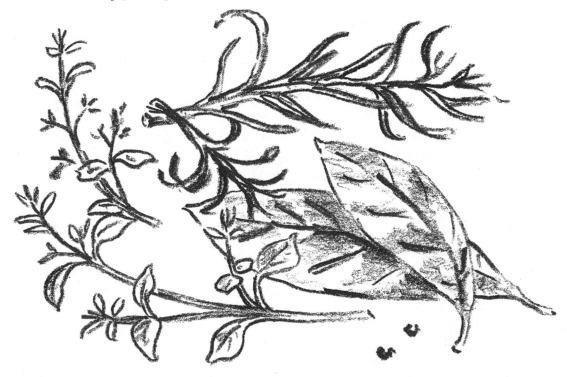

Raspberry Curd____

Makes 450g/1 lb

UK

225g/8 oz raspberries
100g/4 oz caster sugar
2 × size 2 eggs plus 2 extra yolks
50g/2 oz butter

US

1½ cups raspberries
½ cup superfine sugar
2 large eggs plus 2 extra yolks
¼ cup butter

1. Crush raspberries in a large heatproof bowl, then whisk in sugar.
2. Beat in eggs and extra yolks.
3. Add butter, cut into small pieces.
4. One quarter fill a saucepan with hot water. Place on stove. Rest bowl of mixture over saucepan without allowing water to touch bowl.
5. Cook over low heat, stirring continuously until curd thickens.
6. Pour through a nylon sieve into a large jug [this is to remove seeds], then pour into a serving bowl if using the same day or pot in jam jars, sealing in the usual way. Store for up to one week.

Use in place of lemon curd for spreads or cake fillings.

C
W
D — if vegetable margarine substituted
Veg

Migraine Sufferer's Diary

Time of getting up and going to bed	Bowel Movement	Food	Beverages	Weather	Social and Work Activity
6 a.m.					
7					
8					
9					
10					
11					
12					
1 p.m.					
2					
3					
4					
5					
6					
7					
8					
9					
10					
11					
12					

Reproduced from the Migraine Trusts *A Pocket Guide for Migraine Sufferers*

News	Extra Travel	Extra Exercise	Medication	Menstrual Cycle	Migraine

BIBLIOGRAPHY

The Allergy Cookbook Ruth Shattuck [Century Publishing, 1985]

Allergy Self-help Cookbook Marjorie Hurt Jones, RN [Rodale Press, 1984]

Answers to Migraine F Clifford Rose and Paul Davies [Macdonald, 1987]

Composition of Foods McCance and Widdowson (HMSO)

Dictionary of Nutrition and Food Technology Arnold E Bender [Newnes Butterworth]

Food Allergy P Scowen [Edsall, 1985]

Food of the Western World Theodora Fitzgibbon [Hutchinson]

Food Intolerance Robert Buist [Prism Press, 1984]

Gluten-free Cooking Rita Greer [Thorsons Publishing Group, 1983]

Mastering Your Migraine Peter Evans [Grafton, 1988]

The Headache Book Edda Hanington [Technomic Publishing]

Migraine Edda Hanington [Priory Press]

Migraine — The Facts F Clifford Rose and M Gawel [OUP, 1981]

The Role of Tyramine in the Aetiology of Migraine E Hanington and A M Harper

Understanding Migraine [Migraine Trust]

Useful Contacts

Australia/New Zealand

The names of individual clinics can be
  acquired from patient's doctors

Belgium

Belgian Migraine Society,
  Konigslaan 17,
  B-2340 Beerse

Canada

The Migraine Foundation,
  390 Brunswick Avenue,
  Toronto,
  Ontario M5R 224

Denmark

Scandinavian Migraine Association,
  Sandrz A/S Liniskforskningsad,
  Tilangade 9A,
  DK2200,
  Kobenhavn N

West Germany

International Headache Society,
  Klinikum Grobhadern,
  NRO-Poliklinik,
  Marchionistrasse 15,
  8000 Munchen 70

United Kingdom

The Migraine Trust,
  45 Great Ormond Street,
  London WC1N 3HD

British Migraine Association,
  178A High Road,
  Byfleet,
  Surrey

United States of America

The American Association for the Study
  of Headache,
  5252 N Western Avenue,
  Chicago,
  Illinois 60625

National Headache Association,
  5252 North Western Avenue,
  Chicago,
  Illinois 60625

American Pain Society,
  340 Kingsland St,
  Nutley,
  New Jersey 07110

INDEX

C – citrus free; D – dairy free; MSG – Monosodium glutamate free;
Veg – vegetarian; Vegan – vegan; W – wheat free

THE MIGRAINE REVOLUTION

Dr John Mansfield

Over 5 million people in the UK alone suffer from migraine at some time in their lives. The incidence is higher in women than in men and estimates have suggested that approximately 20 per cent of the adult female population suffers from this condition at some point.

Now, after countless trials conducted all over the world, it has been concluded that food allergy is *the* main single cause of migraine — accounting for between 80 and 95 per cent of cases. The foods involved are quite diverse, but the most persistent offenders are such common foods as wheat, corn, milk, sugar and oranges.

Dr John Mansfield explores the factors underlying the occurrence of allergy, pointing the way to a healthier lifestyle and eating habits which will lessen the chance of continued migraine attacks. He shows why allergic manifestations occur at certain times in a person's life and why people may be able to eat commonly-consumed foods for many years before an adverse reaction sets in.

As Dr Mansfield says, 'This new approach to illness, which is best termed clinical ecology, is in my view the most exciting development in medicine since the discovery of antibiotics . . . This has become truly a total revolution in the treatment of migraine.'